To

The Power of the Past

Nice to get
to know you, I
Hope we will talk
again.

The Power of the Past

*Transformational Replay
Regression Therapy*

Drake Eastburn, BCH, CI

Contents

Foreword

As a hypnotherapist and instructor, I am gratified to see this work in print. The use of regression in hypnosis is one of the most valuable elements available to us as therapists, and it is enormously beneficial to our clients as well. Yet it can also be the most feared and misunderstood. I have had the opportunity to train Certified Hypnotherapists in the advanced methods of HypnoFertility and Gestalt-based Hypnotherapy, which routinely employ regression work. While many hypnotherapists are comfortable with hypnotic regression, many more are not, and some, perhaps because of misunderstanding the process, have avoided integrating it into their practice. Because of my firm belief in its power, I include an overview of Drake's regression technique, Transformational Replay, in all the programs I teach. I have found that students, once they have become comfortable with it, repeatedly praise it as the most comprehensive regression instruction they have ever received.

There truly is power in accessing the past, and a properly done regression is unequalled in the realm of rapid-change therapy. While it is not a panacea, neither is regression something that should be avoided or feared by a properly trained hypnotherapist. In the therapeutic repertoire of someone like Drake Eastburn, its value is inestimable. I can honestly say that I have never met a better or more knowledgeable hypnotherapist than Drake. He is intuitive and insightful, and his expertise and skill, wisdom and humor illuminate every page of this book. His rich and varied experience in hypnosis reaches back more than 30 years. Other hypnotherapists have often expressed the desire to be a fly on the wall in Drake's private sessions. This book is their chance.

World-renowned author, lecturer and advanced instructor Roy Hunter, M.S., has singled out Eastburn Institute of Hypnosis graduates as some of the best-trained students he has ever had the pleasure to teach, remarking on their ability to grasp the concepts and value of regression. Many of our graduates have expressed appreciation as well for the depth and breadth of the education they received from us, particularly with regard to the regression component of our curriculum, and especially after meeting other hypnotists who trained elsewhere.

After practicing many years in the field of hypnosis, and having attended and taught numerous basic and advanced trainings, I have yet to encounter a more effective regression method than that which Drake teaches. And I know of no one else who presents regression as he presents it. I encourage you to apply Drake's technique to your own practice, and see for yourself just how effectively and efficiently you can assist your clients in experiencing resolution and healing.

LYNSI EASTBURN, BCH, CI

Arvada, Colorado
November 9, 2006

Acknowledgments

Thanks go out to all of those who have supported me in my hypnosis journey. My wife, Lynsi, has created a huge name for herself in the world of hypnosis in a very short time. She amazes me with her ability to understand the principles of hypnosis and therapy and apply them as only she could. Her grasp of the English language and the mechanics involved help me to appear better than I really am. Having the two of us working so hard in this field at the same time has given us an advantage that few other hypnotherapists have.

Martie O'Brien is our beloved office manager and, along with Philo Couch, was instrumental in creating the graphics for this book. I rely on her editorial skills constantly. The support that she gives so freely is no small contribution to getting a project like this accomplished and keeping Eastburn Hypnotherapy running.

Many thanks to long-time friend and colleague, Anita DiStefano, who dropped everything to help put the finishing touches on this book and who also provided the typesetting.

Thanks to Jerry Kein and Omni Hypnosis for the use of the Hypnosis Mind Model. (See "References" in the back for more about Jerry Kein and Omni Hypnosis.)

I would like to give a special thanks to the late Jerry Haskins. Jerry and I met in a hypnosis class about thirty years ago. It was

Jerry's dream to become a hypnotherapist. While Jerry and I did a lot of hypnosis together he never made that shift into making a living as a hypnotherapist. He was supportive of me every step of the way and proofread a lot of my earlier material. Jerry would be thrilled with how things have developed.

Introduction

The information in this book will be of great interest to a wide variety of individuals. The portion of the book that outlines using therapeutic methods is meant for trained hypnotherapists only. If you are a hypnotherapist, but possess few skills in this area, I suggest getting proper training prior to attempting these methods. We do offer such training. Other than Gerry Kein, Steven Parkhill, or my wife, Lynsi Eastburn, there are few others that I know of with whom I would recommend training, although that's not to say there aren't others who may be qualified. Unfortunately, many therapists are doing only pseudo-regressions, likely because that is how they were trained.

I am a big fan of therapy in general. I have experienced a wide variety of therapies myself and have trained in various methods such as Gestalt Therapy, Rational Emotive Behavioral Therapy, Thought Field Therapy, Eye Motion Desensitization and Reprocessing, Emotional Freedom Technique and various methods of Hypnotherapy. Hypnotherapy seems to me to be, by far, the quickest and most successful method in most cases. Certainly there are issues that may not be appropriate for hypnosis. While we can deal with grief through hypnosis, I also recommend that people see a qualified grief counselor. Grief counselors possess skills in this area that can be very helpful during someone's time of need. Hypnosis can be helpful with relationship issues as well; however, a good relationship counselor can be worth his or her weight in gold. While I am of the opinion that it is best if we can solve things without the use of medication, there are times when medication is absolutely necessary. The modality someone is trained in (that is, their profession) may color how he or she sees each client. If you are a hammer then you tend to see the world as a nail. If you take your issue to an acupuncturist, then he or she will see you as a place to put needles. If you go to a chiropractor, then you become a potential for adjustment. A medical doctor might see you as something to cut open and repair or to put medications into. Whatever method we may choose to work with should not blind us to other possibilities. I never hesitate to refer someone for some other type of work if it appears necessary. People come to me all the time with stress and stiff muscles and obviously hypnosis is helpful and so is a massage.

Often people seem to avoid seeking help for emotional needs, due to the stigma around mental health issues. If someone receives a diagnosis, it can often be detrimental, because the diagnosis could follow us around through insurance and employment history. We need to get over this antiquated thinking surrounding emotional issues. We live in a very fast-paced, high stress world, and we need to be able to seek out professional help. Things will happen to us all at some point or another. A family member could die unexpectedly, or a relationship or career could end. We can and should receive help for these issues. If we fail to get help, the discomfort may continue for a period of time much longer than necessary. Other issues may have been plaguing us since Day One and these things can be dealt with as well. If a person receives benefit—regardless of the type of therapy they choose—then that's a good thing.

If, after reading this book, you feel you are someone who could benefit from this type of therapy, you will need to seek out a proper hypnotherapist. A good place to start would be through the National Guild of Hypnotists. The NGH is the largest and oldest certifying body of its kind and they can provide you with names of therapists in your area.

Talk to more than one therapist before deciding on someone. Make certain your therapist seems confident. If they say things like, this *might* work or we could *try* to help you, then they are not very confident. At Eastburn Hypnotherapy Center we offer a free half-hour consultation. This can be very personal work and I believe people should have an opportunity to meet their therapist face to face and make sure that they click. I suggest choosing a therapist who practices hypnotherapy as their main modality. A person becomes a good hypnotherapist by doing hypnotherapy over and over, day after day. Many licensed mental health people have only had a short course in hypnosis and only use hypnosis as an adjunct to their other work. However, having a degree in some other modality doesn't make you a great hypnotherapist; it's doing the work consistently that makes you good at hypnotherapy.

What is the benefit from the type of therapy presented in this book? Lots of different types of issues, such as phobias (very common), anxiety, a wide variety of emotional issues, weight (that doesn't respond to other work), can be dealt with through this type of regression therapy. I don't usually look at regression as being the first line of work to do with someone. In fact, as time has gone on, I do less regression, because I have developed other methods that I use first. At the Eastburn clinics we usually start with the easiest methods, such as suggestion work. If a client runs up against blocks then we are more likely to pursue regression. When I work with phobias, I usually start off with regression because phobias can shift so quickly.

We no longer live in a world where we have to accept or stay stuck in whatever issue may be plaguing us. Nor do we live in a world where we must spend years resolving those issues. So we must each ask ourselves: *How good am I willing to have it?*

1

How We Become Who We Are

I'm a big fan of some of the Zen-like philosophies of "living in the moment." Certain books that I have read, such as *Be Here Now, Chop Wood, Carry Water* or *The Power of Now*, are big proponents of this *in the present* kind of living. Certainly, we are not in the moment nearly enough. Some of that is, of course, due to our life-in-the-fast-lane style of living. The current cliché, *just get over it,* may be the modern version of *be in the moment.*

I am an avid student in the field of genetics and believe that, now that the genetic code has recently been broken, we can expect to see huge breakthroughs coming our way. New books are coming out all the time and soon genetics will be, more and more, a common topic on the tongues of everyday people. It is well documented that we are pre-programmed through our genes, and this has more to do with who we are and how we respond to what goes on in our world than anything else. Some people are appalled by this notion. Why would someone like me, who is in the nurture business, be looking so intensely at our hardwiring?

While our genetic makeup does play a huge role, the genes don't limit us to a single option. The same person subjected to a harsh arctic climate will respond differently to a tropical climate. Everyone probably experiences depression at some time in his or her life. Some people may have a genetic propensity towards depression; however, if the circumstance that would cause the feelings of depression to arise never occurs, then those genes do not respond. There are people walking around in the world today who have the alcoholic gene, yet they are not alcoholics, simply because they aren't doing the one thing that would trigger that gene into action. That is to say, they just don't drink. I think we can probably all agree that *the flight or fight response* is something that we are all programmed with. Yet we don't run around all day long in fight or flight—there needs to be some cause for it to occur. Some genes do nothing but trigger other genes. We respond genetically based to a great degree on our environment (nurture).

While I love the whole *be in the moment* philosophy, I just don't believe it's so. In any given moment not much is really going on and whatever is going on is a product of all the history that occurred prior to that moment. Even the thought that I am in the moment is a product of the history that led to the moment. Without our history there would be no moment.

If we relate it to music, the now is just one single note. No matter how sweet that note might sound for that brief moment while it's drifting through the air, it is just one brief note. It is all the other notes that led up to that note that create the melody (history) that, when brought together, sounds so delicious. With only one note there will be no melody and symbols can never crash and we will never experience the crescendo.

Our history creates the melody of our lives. Without our history we would not be the people we are today. Each moment in our lives is one of the notes that creates the melody (story) of our lives. And it's all of those events that eventually create the crescendo of our lives.

Our history is not a death sentence unless we allow it to be. Our history (circumstances) can be an excuse (justification) or a reason (motivator)—it's up to us. History (the same history) can be the thing that landed us on the Ten Most Wanted list or the Fortune 500 list.

You are, right *now* in this very moment, a product of your history and how you have responded to it. It is my opinion that we are all likely to experience some kind of adversity growing up. Some may seem to get more than their fair share. I believe that we need at least some of these challenges to help us become strong individuals. We need to be met with adversity and work through it. When we have worked through our difficulties in healthy ways, we become stronger as individuals. That's not to say that everyone who has had challenges will be better for it; some people will take their victimization all the way to the grave and never grow from it. (Tune in to the Jerry Springer show some time and see them in action.) People who have had to deal with a lot and have done so in a healthy manner gain wisdom and build character in the process. These are the kinds of people that other people are drawn to for advice and support.

Recognizing our history is only the first step, though probably the most important step, because from there we can begin to move ahead. We can begin to rewrite the symphony of who we are.

The largest barrier to changing our history (or at least how we respond to it) is that the most formative events (core issues) are not normally in our conscious memory. They are, however, in the subconscious memory. For the most part, these formative events occurred by the time we were five years old. This is why traditional cognitive therapy has been so lengthy and only moderately successful. By sitting and talking with the conscious mind, it can take forever to achieve healing in the subconscious. Events that are talked about in cognitive therapy are those events that can be remembered by the conscious mind, and they are not likely to be the cause of a core issue. With Transformational Replay (regression therapy), we can get to the core issue and transform things rather quickly.

2

The "Crucifixion"

I don't know that I had ever told this story to anyone until several years back when I told it to one of my classes to make a point. It worked so well that I've used it with every class ever since. It is a true story. I know because it happened to me.

During the early '70s I had gone away on a three-month-long solo backpacking trip. While hitchhiking through Grand Junction, Colorado, a guy in a pickup truck gave me a lift. He was working as a ranch hand in the Grand Mesa area. He said that he knew of some places to pack into from the ranch that other people weren't likely to know about, so I stayed with him and ended up at the ranch. I helped out with mending fences on the ranch for a day or two and then headed into the backcountry. Spring rains kept me holed up at an old homestead for several days while I waited for a break in the weather. The unseasonably wet spring had washed out access into this area. I wasn't likely to see anyone else; though the ranch hands had told me there were "some crazy Mexican sheepherders" in the high country who would just love to cut up a long-haired hippie like me (thanks for the "suggestion").

I had hiked several days, often through deep snow, and there was never a sign of another human. One morning after I broke camp, I started to head back toward the old, abandoned homestead. I hadn't gone far when I came to an opening in the forest. I could see for a great distance. A long way off was a large hill surrounded by sagebrush and scrub oak. On the top of the hill was what appeared to be a crucifixion! Of course, I thought there was no way that it could be a crucifixion and it was miles away in the distance, so it had to be something else. I could see my journey to the homestead would take me by that hill, so I would be able to take a closer look. From time to time I was getting a little editorial commentary from the back of my mind about those crazy sheepherders.

Occasionally I would break out into a clearing and I could again see the hill way in the distance. Each time it looked more and more like a crucifixion had taken place there, but then that couldn't possibly be, I thought.

Eventually I came out of the forest entirely and was walking through miles and miles of sagebrush and scrub oak. Whenever I got to a high spot I could see the hill and the crucifixion from yet a better vantage point than before. With each improved observation the more convincingly it appeared to be a real crucifixion.

As I approached nearer and nearer to the hill, I found carcasses littering the ground—sheep carcasses in all different states of decomposition. Some of the carcasses had been freshly killed, others were in various stages of decay and others were just bones left bleaching in the sun. One thing was for certain: The closer I got, the more of those dead carcasses littered the ground.

As I started up the hill I could see the crucifixion more and more clearly, but my mind was still telling me, this just can't be. Maybe those crazy sheepherders were nearby. As I moved further and further up the hill it got more and more like one of those bad horror movies where the monster is loose and noises are coming from down in the dark cellar and that dope goes with a flickering match to see if it really is a monster down there. Thoughts were racing through my mind like: *How will I get in touch with the authorities? Will I be able to even get out of here alive?* I was now at a place that, in Gestalt therapy, we refer to as the "choice point." But for me there was no choice, because I was the guy with the flickering match headed down into the dark cellar.

As I got to within about fifty or sixty feet the truth dawned on me: I could see that the crucifixion was actually a scarecrow—a very good scarecrow—but, still, it was only a scarecrow.

What is the point of this story? Simply this: Things aren't always what we think they are. In fact, a lot of what we have based our lives on isn't even real. We go through life as if we are a video camera taking in everything around us through the camera lens (our eyes) with perfect accuracy. There is some truth to this view. But as much as we are the camera recording everything, we are also the projector that is placing the images out there for us to view. What we believe occurs and what actually occurs may not be the same at all.

We operate in paradigms (models) based on our history and beliefs about how the world *should* work. We tend to see the world based on these paradigms, whether they are accurate or not. When a police officer comes to the scene of an accident he/she might get a different version of what happened from each one of the witnesses. All the witnesses saw the same accident, but they all saw it from their own paradigms (expectations). Each one saw it through their own filters. One may have seen that it was a woman driving that blue car and you know she must have been at fault; someone else may have seen that there was a foreign car involved and foreign cars are a problem so that caused the accident. Someone else saw that there was a teenager involved and you know what bad drivers they are, so obviously they must be at fault.

On any street corner the people present are all having different experiences of the same scene. A pickpocket may see everyone else as a possible mark. The person who is alone and on the make may see everyone as a possible partner. The policeman sees everyone as a possible criminal. A beggar may be looking at everyone as a potential donor. The bag lady and the banker are seeing that same street corner through totally different paradigms.

Many years ago I was working for a large school district and I had been called to the scene of an accident to help out. One of our buses had been hit at an intersection by a garbage truck. I helped with some of the children and the driver. Luckily no one was seriously injured. I took many photographs of the scene. Later I was having coffee with my boss and we were talking about the accident. He mentioned that it was such and such kind of a trash truck and I said no, it was one of those ones with the roll off container on the back. My boss was the kind of guy who was always right about everything and would argue forever to prove his point; however, I was so convincing in my description that he thought I must be right. When we got the photographs back I saw that it wasn't the type of truck that I had thought at all, and I was the one taking the pictures at the scene. For whatever reason, my paradigm about what kind of garbage truck runs into school buses was limited and even my being on the scene and photographing the actual event couldn't change that.

What is real? A therapist friend of mine says nothing that happened to us in the past is real. I think that's a little over the top; however, it may be closer to the truth than we think. Certainly if we recall being abused as a youngster we probably were; yet some of the memory of what happened may be more about the memory (based on our paradigms) than what actually may have happened. At that moment on the hill looking at that crucifixion (I referred to it as the "choice point") my reality could have gone many different directions. I could have decided that I could not take even one more step and left and never told anyone what I had seen—in which case, I could have carried the guilt about leaving someone's body hanging on a cross out in the middle of nowhere and it could have eaten away at me forever. I might have chosen to stop at that choice point and go straight to the authorities and report the crucifixion—in which case, I might have ended up sending them on a wild goose chase and feeling like a fool. A number of other possible scenarios come to mind. Would any of these possible scenarios, or the feelings associated with them, not be real? How much of my experience was influenced by the thought in my mind that some crazy, dangerous, sheepherders were lurking about. Any choice I made at that point would have become my reality (along with the emotions and beliefs, associated with that choice). And wouldn't it be real? Believe me, the feelings that are associated with, "Oh my God, it's a crucifixion!" are a lot different than those associated with, "Oh, it's just a scarecrow." All the feelings, all the memories, around any of the possible scenarios involving this scene were real, but only one was accurate.

(Just to clarify, the scarecrow was put on the hill to scare away coyotes. The coyotes were responsible for all of the carcasses lying around. I had run into the sheepherder shortly after my journey up the hill. He was from the Basque region of Spain and was not at all interested in cutting up any long-haired hippies.)

How many times have we created memories about our lives that are real, but not accurate? Have you ever relived a story with others only to find that their interpretation is much different from yours? Who is correct? The fireman arriving at the scene of a home on fire probably has a much different experience of the scenario than the homeowner, or the next-door neighbor, or the insurance agent, or the deliveryman, yet all of their experiences of that scene are valid.

Have you ever leaped from bed in the middle of the night with your heart pounding out of your chest, sweating and out of breath, because you were being chased by a lion or a monster in a dream? Could those feelings have been any more real if there were a lion actually in bed with you? Is the dream real? What is real anyway?

Our belief about what our history is has been instrumental in creating who we are. What if we could just change what we believe to be our reality?

3

Just Make Me Forget

Often people walk into my office and ask me to erase their memory of the whole thing (meaning some uncomfortable situation in their past). Or they will say something like, "I don't remember anything from six to eight years old, and something must have happened, but since I don't remember it, it must not be bothering me."

Wouldn't it be nice if it could be so easy? With hypnosis we could allow someone to forget something; however, the problem with that is we are only forgetting in the conscious mind. Years ago it was a very common practice for hypnotists to suggest that such and such of an uncomfortable nature would not be remembered by the client. However, the reality is that the memory is still in the subconscious mind and we move about in the world as if this thing were occurring all the time.

Forgetting is a strategy that the conscious mind already uses. Often when something happens (a trauma, for instance) the conscious mind will block it out. It helps the individual to get on with life or seemingly erase that part of their history that is too distasteful to deal with. While we have paradigms about how the world should function, we also have paradigms about who we are. If an incident occurs that just doesn't fit into our paradigm about who we are, then we may just block it out.

When I'm interviewing a client I will ask them about the memory of their childhood. Some people have a good memory (fairly complete) of their childhood. For others it is more vague and yet still others have chunks missing. For example: "I don't recall much of anything between six and eight years old." Other people will say, "Why do I only remember the bad stuff?"

The most distinct memories are tied with emotions. It could be any emotion, but the stronger the emotion around the memory the more likely we are to recall it. We will recall things that are associated with enjoyable emotions (falling in love), though the more charge there is (often that means discomfort), the more likely we are to remember an incident. That's why people tend to recall the uncomfortable things that have occurred in their past more readily. When someone says they only have a vague memory of what happened, but no chunks are missing, it is likely that the emotional events that were occurring were not significant enough to cause a strong memory of the times. For example, sitting in front of a Nintendo game for years on end would not likely cause a strong memory of that time period.

The client who has chunks of memory missing is of particular interest to me. I have never journeyed into one of these blank places without uncovering something highly significant. In my experience, journeying into one of these blank spaces has always yielded a positive outcome for the client. Why? Why does it matter what happened in those times if we don't even remember them? The reason is that we do remember them; we just don't remember them consciously. Those memories are a part of our subconscious minds. People often will say, "So what? I live my life normally; there is nothing wrong." And certainly it does seem that way, because we have created coping strategies that allow us to function fairly normally. The problem is we're missing out on the fullest experience of life (we may approach life more as a spectator event). Avoidance is one of our most common coping strategies. We simply do not allow ourselves to be in situations that would make us uncomfortable (seems innocent enough). Each time we avoid something, we are shrinking our experience of life. It doesn't feel like a problem to the person who is avoiding because that situation is uncomfortable anyway. It's easier and more comfortable not to deal with it, and therefore affects our homeostasis (helping us to stay within our comfort zone).

Homeostasis is our body's natural tendency toward good health. We as hypnotherapists can assist this process. Other modalities also assist this process. When a person breaks their arm, the body naturally works to mend the bones. A doctor becomes involved in the process by setting the bone and putting the arm in a cast, thereby enabling the body to achieve its physical homeostasis.

We also have a psychological homeostasis (comfort zone). We can think of our psychological homeostasis like a thermostat on the wall. If you set the thermostat at 70 degrees, the thermostat will signal the furnace to come on if the temperature drops a few degrees. The furnace will shut off once it has reached a temperature a little above 70 degrees. This cycle continues on and on to keep our comfort close to that 70-degree mark. When we participate in coping strategies, we are affecting our homeostasis (comfort zone). The smaller our homeostasis becomes, the smaller our experience of life becomes. What happens when we become slaves to our comfort zone? We don't do things like get on a plane, change our diet, or go for that promotion. Or the weather is too hot or cold or wet to exercise, or we don't become involved in a relationship. Our homeostasis can become so restricted that we will no longer feel comfortable leaving our own home.

People with a much broader homeostasis will have a bigger experience of life and live more fully. They are more likely to go for that promotion, or get involved in an exercise program, or take off on that safari. In fact, they will respond in much healthier ways to traumatic situations, because their experience (paradigms) accepts a greater range of variables.

Years ago I was an ultra distance runner in the mountains of Colorado. I've run many of the fourteen thousand foot peaks there. I've run the Pikes Peak Marathon and the Mount Evans Trophy Run a number of times. During that time in my life I had a grandmother who was a dear, sweet person, but one of those people with a very restricted homeostasis. She was concerned about adjusting window coverings at different times of the day, so that the temperature would always be just so. She always wore dresses with plenty of pockets stuffed with tissues, because you never know when you might need a tissue. She never left the house without at least one sweater. A ride in the car or a trip to Kmart was pushing the extremes of her homeostasis. The first time that I was running the Pikes Peak race, she gave me some of those wet wipe things to put in my pocket in case I might sweat. *In case I might sweat!* I didn't even try to explain that my running shorts didn't have pockets for wet wipes. After the race was over she couldn't even grasp the reality of anyone running on a trail to the top of a fourteen thousand plus peak and back down. In her mind it somehow must be a lot easier than it sounded.

In 1969 the first astronauts landed on the moon. There were a lot of people at that time who said it was fake, it was all done in a Hollywood studio. Their paradigms just did not include people landing on the moon. That's kind of how Grandma saw the Pikes Peak race— it just couldn't be as difficult as it seemed. No one would attempt something like that if it was that difficult. These are extreme examples of the whole homeostasis (comfort zone) piece. Sure, lots of people might have no interest whatsoever in running to the tops of fourteen thousand foot peaks, but just where do you draw that homeostasis line? How big are you willing to live your life?

A lot of times clients come in and they do have some awareness that whatever happened in their past is holding them back in some way. Often they will say, "I know exactly what has caused my problem." Usually they are only aware of those things that are in their conscious memory and not the core event. The important thing is that they have come into my office and now I can help them.

Through *Transformational Replay* we can give the mind a new, more useful scenario to operate from. The memory of the original event will not be erased. Both events are likely to be remembered; however, the mind tends to choose the event that is more beneficial to operate from. Occasionally a client will tell me, "I know what happened and we can't change that." It's the cnscious mind that is saying that and they are right; if we tried to change the conscious mind, it wouldn't work. That's why other modalities haven't done much to resolve their problem.

4

The Inner Child

As part of the Transformational Replay process, the inner child plays a huge role and I must discuss it here. There is a great deal of information available on the inner child. John Bradshaw's work certainly is the most well known. There are many books available by Bradshaw and he travels around the country doing workshops. Most of the work I do in this area has evolved from his work. If you are a hypnotherapist and have not had training in inner child work, I suggest you attend one of Bradshaw's workshops. It will be beneficial to your own healing and the work dovetails nicely with the hypnotic process.

Because so much of what we uncover through the Transformational Replay process has occurred early in life, the child will obviously be involved. Many things can go wrong early in life to create an issue for us later on. Dysfunctional families seem to be the norm anymore; and even in very high functioning families things can go wrong.

When doing an intake with my clients, I ask about any traumas (accidents, surgeries, someone close dying) or abuse (physical, emotional, sexual), especially early in life. Also I ask about their birth experience. Were they on time, late, early, breech, C-section, or the like? Were there any complications with their birth? Were they put in an incubator or kept in a nursery for some reason? Were they breast fed? What was their parents' relationship like during the pregnancy? It's amazing that oftentimes the most important event in our life is something we know little or nothing about. Often the only reason a person does know anything about it is because Mom keeps bringing it up. "I was in labor forty-seven hours with you and you are going to pay for it the rest of your life." While we recount these things jokingly, there is also truth to it.

I have clients who have many problems beginning at the birth experience, and sometimes even in utero. Things like anxiety or abandonment issues often have their roots in the birth experience. A difficult delivery such as the cord being wrapped around the neck, a difficult breech delivery, premature labor, or any number of other possible complications can be the start of anxiety or phobias later in life. Separation from the mother at birth for any number of reasons can be the predecessor of abandonment issues later in life. Bonding with "that woman" is some of the most powerful genetic encoding we possess. In our genetic past if we are not successful at bonding with "that woman," we don't survive. She is our source of nutrients, love and protection. Without bonding with her our survival is doubtful. Even among high functioning, loving, caring parents, it can all too easily go wrong. Sometimes a health emergency arises and the baby is placed in intensive care or must undergo numerous surgeries. These and many other circumstances can interrupt the bonding process. How is that process affected when the mother chooses not to breast feed or if she uses drugs as part of the process? What if the mother has complications and she is taken into surgery? What if the mother has postpartum depression, or the father has left, or the child is just unwanted? What about babies who are born to extremely young, low functioning mothers? This is becoming more and more prevalent of late. What about children of families where there are so many other children that there is not enough of anything for any of them (food, clothes, toys, love, education)? What will the effects of single parent families have on children later on in life? How will children of multiple births, caused by the use of fertility drugs, be affected later in life?

It's nothing new that adopted children have more issues. It makes sense given what I've been talking about. I'm a huge advocate of adoption and I think people who adopt children are doing a wonderful thing for everyone involved and the world in general. I do not, however, think that it will necessarily be a bed of roses. Certainly, a lot of adopted children move out into the world and do just fine, and that's wonderful. Those who have more difficulty would be well served by the Transformational Replay process and inner child work.

What are some of the main ways that a baby comes to be?

- If we have a baby it will bring us closer together.
- A baby will allow me to feel loved.
- By becoming pregnant I can trap this person into a relationship.
- By getting this person pregnant I can trap them into a relationship.
- I've always wanted to name a boy "Joe Jr." after myself.
- If I have children I can stay at home and I won't have to get a real job.
- It was your turn to go the drug store.
- There was a power failure.
- I'm not cut out for college.
- All of my friends are having babies and I want one too.
- God wants us to procreate.
- I'm getting older and if I don't have a baby now it may become too late.
- I've always dreamt of naming a child Boniface.

- We need a labor force.
- Babies are so cute.
- No men seem to want to get in a committed relationship with me, so I'll just get pregnant anyway.
- My parents were lousy parents; I'm going to show them how it's done.
- My grandmother had twelve kids and she was an amazing woman and I want to be just like her.
- We can afford it now, so we might as well have a kid.
- I thought if he pulled out I wouldn't get pregnant.
- If I get pregnant now, I could have a Pisces!
- My company (or government) is offering a great maternity leave program and I need to take advantage of it right now while it's still available.
- He said he had a condom.
- I am not too young to become a parent and I'm going to prove it.
- I loved playing with my Barbies as a little girl.
- We're going to keep trying until we have a girl (boy).
- We need a boy to carry on the Jones' name.
- I'm allergic to cats.
- Bobby was the cutest and most popular boy in school and I had to put out or he wouldn't date me.
- Another child will increase the size of my welfare check.
- I don't want to be alone.
- I promised Mom I would give her grandchildren.
- We were using the rhythm method.
- This never happened before.
- Oooops.

In my view, bringing another human being into this world should never just be an oooops decision. Ideally, it should be a well thought out, well planned process prior to conception. The process would begin with two high functioning, highly compatible individuals who are truly in love. People are making a choice that will affect them for the rest of their lives and, more importantly, will affect the life of that child. The child doesn't even get to have a say in the one decision that will be the most profound decision ever made in regard to him or her.

Often we hear people say that if you're having an abortion, then you are playing God, but aren't we playing God anyway? Isn't the decision about coming into this world every bit as important as the one to exit? Yet rarely do we confront anyone about his or her choice to become pregnant. Other than in some instances of rape, we have the ability to make that choice.

Our genetic programming around procreation is very powerful; if it were not, we would fail to survive as a species. Through evolution we have also gained a great ability to reason—more so than any other species—and perhaps we could use that more. It's likely that you can look out a window nearby and see buildings or roadways or other man-made structures. The point is it's difficult to look in any direction and not see the effects humans have had on the land. We do not need more bodies to keep the species going. We are in little danger of disappearing, yet we continue to procreate as if we would disappear. We already feel the effects of large population. The process of becoming a family needs to become healthier.

My wife, Lynsi, is probably the foremost authority in the area of hypnosis for fertility. It's a pleasure to see people coming in to see her, because I know that they have been considering the issue of becoming parents for a long time before they came to her office. Most people do not give becoming a parent that kind of thought. If everyone had given the process that much thought I could gaze out my window onto a vast prairie with herds of buffalo roaming over great distances—presuming, that is, that I was around and had a window!

Even if we are wanted and planned for, and born into a family with good loving parents, things can still go bad. In the not so distant past babies were treated as if they had no ability to feel or experience any of the process of birth. Parents and doctors are becoming more aware of the importance of a gentle birth. Methods like Hypno-Birthing® help to insure a more natural, easy birthing process. Through my experience with the Transformational Replay process, I am convinced that these early experiences are formative in how we experience life later on.

As we grow up, it's important that we are able to just be kids. Too often children miss out on that opportunity. It's an important part of our development. There are many reasons why we might miss out on being children. Oftentimes, if there are lots of children in the family, the older kids will have to act as parents, taking care of their younger siblings and missing out on their own childhood. Other times, children have to become responsible early because their parents aren't parenting, because they are alcoholics or drug addicts. Perhaps it's a poor family and the parents are busy working several jobs to pay the bills and keep food on the table, and the children have to take adult responsibilities. Maybe the parents have psychological problems, or are just plain irresponsible. Some children, with otherwise high functioning parents, have to take on adult responsibilities due to language barriers. People migrate from other countries and have difficulty learning the language, but children pick up on languages quite quickly and, as a result, they end up taking care of business dealings, answering phone calls, paying the bills, and negotiating with the landlord. Similar situations may occur if a parent were to become handicapped. Once they become adults, these children may evolve into workaholics because that's what they know. They may have trouble being happy and carefree and playful as adults. They are likely not to find the joy in life as easily as others. They may resent their siblings later on because they missed out on so much.

What if it's a lot worse? What if the child was abused physically, emotionally or sexually? Perhaps they were told they were stupid or ugly, or that they are the cause of the problems in the family (or the world).

One of the things that shapes our self worth is what the rest of the world reflects back to us. If we keep hearing things like, "You're smart, you're talented, you're athletic, you're pretty," then we tend to think of ourselves in that way. What if the messages we got were that we aren't worth anything? Our self worth is then reflected from the world back to us. If we continually received the message that we were stupid over and over from our parents, then some well meaning teacher along the way will have a difficult time overriding all of that previous conditioning.

Many times a beautiful, young woman has come into my office thinking that she's ugly and worthless, because her sister was always presented as the smart, pretty one. Some parents use a critical style of parenting, rarely complementing the child's achievements, and instead always pointing out what's wrong. With some parents nothing will ever be good enough. If you want to raise children who become compulsive or perfectionists, that's a good way to go about it.

Children are not born into this world as evil, or with duties or guilt. The child is born into the world perfect and innocent. The new child has not yet formed a critical mind and is therefore receptive to whatever information they are presented with as the truth.

Children view themselves as the center of their world. If things happen to be going wrong in their world, then somehow they believe they are the cause of it. Let's say that Mommy and Daddy are having a big fight and little Suzy is watching or hears it from the next room. It's easy for us as adults to understand that sometimes parents do fight, but Suzy is thinking something more like, "Things are bad; Mommy and Daddy are screaming; there must be something wrong with me. If only I was a better little Suzy, this wouldn't be happening." The implication is that there must be something inherently wrong with me (which only serves to create shame). Later on in life when the critical mind is more fully formed, little Suzy can observe things differently. Now when Mommy and Daddy are arguing she can see the dynamics of what just happened: Daddy did that, and then Mommy said that, and then Daddy got loud, and Mommy threw something. Now Suzy can see how she is separate from all of their interaction.

Children tend to make decisions around these emotional situations and these decisions are designed to protect us at the time; however, they may come back to bite us later. Let's say that little Suzy is Daddy's little girl and they are really tight. The fighting between Mommy and Daddy leads to a divorce and Daddy is forever out of the picture. As a result little Suzy is left heartbroken. She makes a decision that if you ever love a man he will leave so she decides she will never love a man again. For the time being, this decision may serve her. (God help any stepfather that might come along.) Worse yet, how about when she becomes a young woman? Forming relationships with men would then be a normal part of life. She may find herself subconsciously sabotaging herself or only becoming involved with men who are unavailable. Here we have an adult life being dictated by the decisions of a four-year-old.

When parents themselves are injured children, there's a high likelihood that they will not make good parents. Often they will be looking to get their own needs met and the child will suffer as a result. Some parents look to their child to be an adult to them, to advise and support them. (That is the way that my parents were with me.) Some children seem to have an innate ability to provide that sort of support; however, aren't they being put in a very adult role? The child's role should not be about responsibility.

Many years ago my older brother and I built three canoes. We went on a trip down the Colorado River, from a place called Cisco Pump in Utah near the Colorado border, to Moab, Utah. My brother was in a canoe by himself, my dad and nephew were in another canoe, and my ex-wife and I were in my canoe.

It was a pretty easy float for several days. One morning we were shoving off from shore along with some rafters. Usually my ex-wife and I were out ahead, but this morning we got off to a slow start and everyone was well ahead of us. I was watching down river when I saw the heads of the rest of our party drop out of sight, signifying white water ahead. I yelled at my ex to get her life jacket on. We were prepared as we entered the huge drop in the river.

At the bottom of the rapids I could see my brother paddling around frantically. My nephew was off to my right on some high ground that he had made his way to. Off to my left was a cliff with a large split in the rock and I could see my dad up there in that split. We made it through the rapids, but had taken on a great deal of water. The other members of our party were out of my brother's field of vision and once I let him know that everyone was safe, he could begin gathering stray gear that was floating about the river. While my ex was working at bailing out the canoe, I went about the task of getting my father out of the split in the rocks.

An amazing thing had occurred to me when we were floating through the middle of those rapids. When I looked over to the left and saw my father, he had a forlorn, scared look about him. It was as if he were saying, "Daddy, Daddy, save me." It dawned on me that at that moment I was the parent and he was the child. From then on our relationship took a huge shift and I've never viewed him the same since.

I worked my way through the rapids edging along the cliff wall until I got to the split in the rock. Dad was obviously terrified and was relieved that I had gotten to him. He was just a scared little child and "Daddy" was there to save him. I told him we needed to jump out into the rapids and let the water carry us downstream to the others. He was afraid and said that he couldn't do it. I told him, "Hey, there's no McDonalds or Wal-Mart here; you can't live in a crack in the rock!" He said the current here wouldn't let you float downstream; it would just wash you right back into the crack. I jumped in the rapids to see and, sure enough, the eddy current was too strong and wouldn't allow us to float down. I told him the only thing we could do would be to work our way back along the cliff wall through the rapids, the same way that I had just come. I took hold of him and made him feel safer and eventually we were successful at getting out. From then on, there was an unspoken understanding about who the parent was and who the child was.

Some years later when Mom passed away, Dad would come and stay with me for the summers. I always related to him as the child and he responded to that well. It was easy for me to see him as the injured child that he was since early in his life. I didn't have great expectation for him to perform as a father. My older brother never could get to that place and kept looking toward Dad to provide all the things a dad might provide. But he always met with disappointment. For many years they wouldn't speak to one another—or if they did, it ended badly. Eventually each took his own life.

It's an illusion that we grow up. Mostly we just get larger. Who we are is pretty well formed by the time we're five years old. Nothing magical occurs the day we graduate, or get married, or join the army. We still get jealous of the one who has the newest or most toys; they're just bigger and more expensive now. Sometimes, as we get older, we forget to play; people just aren't silly enough; we take life too seriously.

When was the last time you went to a playground to swing on the swings? Do you remember how it felt to swing as high as you could go and point your toes up to the sky and lean way back and look at the ground rushing towards you? It's hard to take yourself too seriously when your stomach is up in your throat and you're squealing with excitement. What if we took that little five-year-old kid that's in all of us to work with us? What if, as couples, we allowed ourselves to interact as kids and allowed ourselves to be more playful?

We walk around in our five-foot-nine-inch world of mono-vision, missing out on a whole lot. Try looking at the world from the point of view of a little kid. Little kids are down there close to the ground exploring every little detail of life. They're curious about every creepy, crawly thing in the grass. When a kid gets by a stream or a pond, they get up close and personal with the pollywogs and water bugs. Kids don't mind getting dirty and wet, and the feel of mud oozing between their toes is a fun thing. As grownups we're all concerned about keeping our clothes neat and clean and being appropriate.

If the child part of us is injured, then we may find ourselves being held back. For example, when we have the skills and knowledge to go for that promotion, but we feel ourselves being too afraid to move ahead, often it's the child who is holding us back. The adult part of us knows we can do it: "After all, I have a master's degree and twelve years of experience in the field; there's no reason why I shouldn't go for that promotion." The problem isn't the adult. The adult part does have the capability; it's the child part of us that's afraid. This situation just feels too similar to some other scary thing that happened before. When we bond with and comfort the child, the child then feels safe and the adult can move ahead.

Children who participated in extracurricular activities like sports, drama, music, choir, and whose parents were there on the sidelines cheering them on, tend to do better later in life. Even when little Johnny falls and misses the score at the soccer game, Mom or Dad is there to pick him up, brush him off and send him back into the game. These kids do better later in life. They tend to see the world as a safer place and, even if they fail, things will be okay (even though Mommy and Daddy are not around). These are the kids who later in life will go for that promotion, or write that book, or set out on that business venture.

Children who are raised by parents who aren't supportive or have a more critical parenting style may find themselves feeling less safe moving ahead later in life.

When I was in Junior High and High School I went out for wrestling. I was strong and athletic, but I never did all that well. There were times when I was out on the mat and I knew I was better than my opponent and I could easily beat him, yet I just didn't have that little bit of extra drive that it took to win. My good friend, Bob, wrestled on our team in Junior High one season. He was a very big, tall kid. He was way taller than anyone else in school. He had long, gangly arms and legs and was awkward and clumsy and geeky and anything but an athlete.

He was the heavyweight wrestler on our team; in fact, he was probably the only kid that we had who could wrestle heavy weight. In any of the other weight classes you always knew that you would be wrestling someone within about ten pounds of your own weight; however, in the heavyweight division anything goes and one wrestler could be significantly outmatched. Oftentimes Bob was faced with a monster out on the mat. I'd seen Bob walk out on the mat and trip over his own feet and fall on his face and he and the crowd got a big laugh about it. Then he would go on to beat his opponent. In fact, Bob never lost a match. He didn't have any style, or athletic ability. Some of the things that happened on the mat were laughable, but he always won his match.

What was the big difference between Bob and me? The difference was that Bob's dad was always on the sidelines. In those days there were no video cameras, but Bob's dad had one of those old cameras that you had to keep winding up all the time to shoot home movies. Bob Senior was always on the sidelines cheering his son on and getting the rest of the crowd excited and involved. I could see this was the big difference—my friend, Bob, had support—he had his own cheering squad. This was true on or off the mat. Bob's dad was always supportive of him in all areas. Bob was never a great student, but he did really well in life. He built up a number of businesses even at a very young age and was always successful in his endeavors—all because of the encouragement he got earlier in life.

Bob's world was in sharp contrast to mine. The only reason I got to wrestle was because it didn't cost anything. Musical instruments were out of the question, due to cost. It wasn't so much that we couldn't afford those things, but they were just very low on my parents' list of priorities. No one even bothered to ask how I was doing on the wrestling team (it just wasn't important). My older brother had gone out for football. Years later, he said that Mom or Dad had never come to any of his games. I said, "Damn! That's great to know! I thought it was just me that they didn't care about!"

Nowadays I enjoy going to my two stepsons' events. They both are playing musical instruments and that's great. I enjoyed cheering them on when they were playing roller hockey. Even though I work a very busy schedule, I try to make time for all of their events. It's better than making excuses later.

The Inner Child Journey

Often I will do a hypnosis session that enables my clients to meet their inner child. This is often done as a separate session prior to a Transformational Replay or other kinds of hypnotic work. A protocol for this process is included later on in this book, should you be a therapist who wants to take advantage of this process.

5

The Hypnosis Mind Model

T he mind model on the following pages fits in with the inner child and the rest of the work that we will be dealing with here. I am presenting this mind model as I have learned it from Jerry Kein and Steven Parkhill (see Figure 1).

In the center of our mind model you can see we have the *unconscious mind*, which is made up of the nervous system. Basically, these are the functions of the body that we don't normally control consciously. We can and do control them at times; for example, we can regulate our breathing or affect our heart rate and blood pressure rather easily just by using our own thoughts. However, for the most part we are not conscious of these functions as we go about our daily lives.

The next portion of the diagram is the circle that surrounds the unconscious mind and that is the *subconscious mind*. To a hypnotherapist this is the area of the mind that we are most focused upon. This is the area that contains our long-term and permanent memory, emotions, habits and self-preservation.

The outer circle is the *conscious mind*. The conscious mind contains our short-term memory. It contains our willpower, and analytical, critical, rational, and judgmental kinds of thinking.

Figure 1
HYPNOSIS AND THE MIND MODEL*

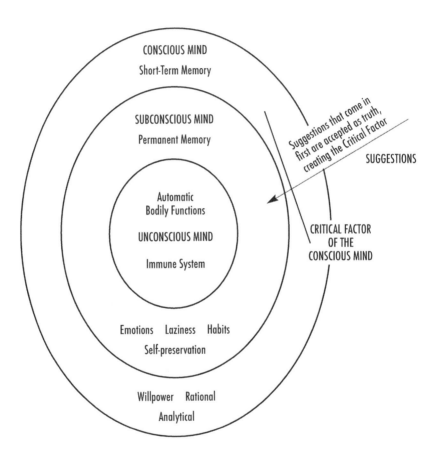

Hypnosis is the bypass of the Critical Factor of the Conscious Mind
and the establishment of acceptable selective thinking.

*By Gerald F. Kein.

While we are infants, the subconscious mind is wide open and accepts any input that comes in as if it's the truth. If we are told that a circle is a square and we hear that over and over again, then that becomes the truth for us. Later on, if we are told that the circle is not a square, it may be difficult for us to change our thinking. This belief that a circle is really a square becomes accepted as truth and becomes part of our *critical factor*. The critical factor (referred to as the *critical faculty* by Dave Elman) is really there to protect us against detrimental input. The critical factor becomes like a shield, and any information that comes in that is not consistent with the critical factor is deflected. We take in a lot of information very quickly when we're young, and it's necessary that we receive information this way. But the problem is that not all of those early messages that help to form the critical factor are good for us. The example of a circle being a square is a simple one.

Throughout this text I may use the terms "critical factor" or "critical faculty" interchangeably and this has become common practice in the field. The term "critical faculty," however, is probably the correct usage.

What if the early input was not so good? Let's say that the early input was that we were unwanted, or we were ugly, or worthless, or stupid. As a result, we go through our lives through the filter of being unwanted, ugly, worthless, or stupid. It's not hard to see how this type of input to the critical factor could cripple us to some extent. Later on, as we receive better input, that new good input is rejected by our critical factor. Pity the poor teacher who sees potential in a young child, yet can't seem to get through to them.

As you can see in Figures 2 and 3, when a strong critical factor has been created around negative input, the positive suggestions just bounce off.

Ideally, we would receive positive information in early life that would help to create a positive critical faculty such as the one in Figure 4. Receiving that positive input early on helps to ensure confidence and high self-esteem later in life. When our critical faculty has been built up around the input of positive reinforcement, our

Figure 2
HYPNOSIS AND THE MIND MODEL*

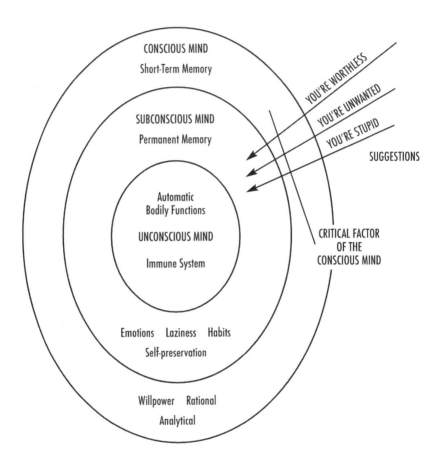

Hypnosis is the bypass of the Critical Factor of the Conscious Mind and the establishment of acceptable selective thinking.

*By Gerald F. Kein.

Figure 3
HYPNOSIS AND THE MIND MODEL*

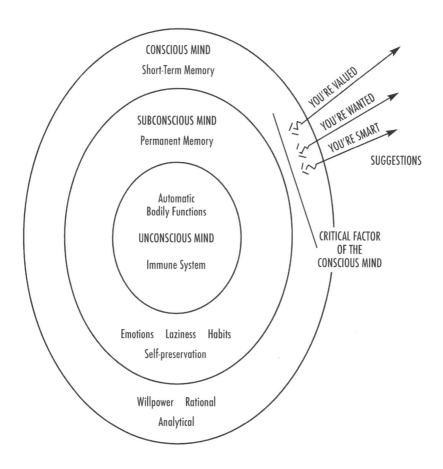

Hypnosis is the bypass of the Critical Factor of the Conscious Mind and the establishment of acceptable selective thinking.

*By Gerald F. Kein.

Figure 4
HYPNOSIS AND THE MIND MODEL*

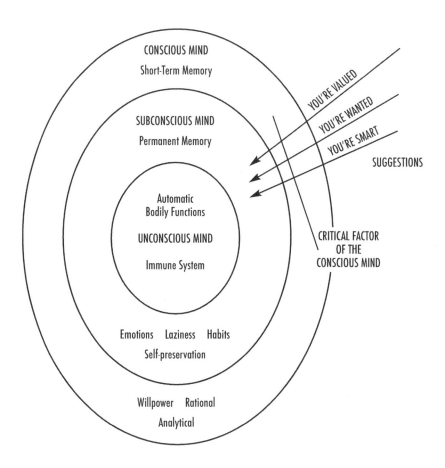

Hypnosis is the bypass of the Critical Factor of the Conscious Mind and the establishment of acceptable selective thinking.

*By Gerald F. Kein.

self-esteem will be none the worse for wear when negative information comes in. The new negative information will come up against the critical faculty and just bounce off.

Can we change the critical factor? The good news is yes. Will it be easy? That depends on how much went into forming the critical factor in the first place. The more we get the same kind of input into the critical factor and the more emotion there is around it, the stronger it becomes. The belief that the circle is really a square could probably change fairly easily if there is not a lot of emotional trauma connected with it. All of the input from the rest of the world that says squares are squares and circles are circles, may be enough to change that part of the critical factor. What went into forming the critical factor in the first place determines how much it will take to change it. Doing affirmations over and over can break down that critical factor and change our attitudes. It may even be possible to break through some really strong conditioning with just affirmations; however, one may need to be endlessly relentless to achieve such success.

Being led to believe that a circle is a square is a lot different from being told you're worthless or ugly or stupid while you're being abused. Like I said earlier, memory that is associated with strong emotions is memory that sticks with us the most and forms a stronger critical factor.

Hypnotherapy is directed at the subconscious mind. In hypnosis, the critical factor is "softened" and easier to get through. In this softening of the critical factor, suggestions can go right into the subconscious mind and create changes. Other times we can achieve a complete bypass of the critical factor and the subconscious receives suggestions (changes) directly. This is what often occurs in the Transformational Replay process. There are many ways in which a hypnotherapist might bypass the critical factor.

At our clinic we generally start work with the easiest methods first. If we can resolve an issue without doing regression work, it's much easier for everyone. If we run into barriers, then regression is usually necessary.

6

How It All Happens

Early on, an incident occurs which we'll call a trauma. Perhaps it's some sort of birth experience. That incident by itself could end up being nothing of great consequence. However, if another incident follows that is similar to that first incident, or at least has the same kind of emotions attached to it, then that first incident becomes more meaningful. Any other incident of the same kind or with the same emotions connected with it only serves to compound that first incident (actually the emotions associated with it). The first incident is now what we refer to as the ISE, or Initial Sensitizing Event. The events that follow help to compound the ISE and are called SSEs, or Subsequent Sensitizing Events. There can be a great many SSEs.

Let's just say, for example, that a difficult birth produced feelings of anxiety or abandonment for little Suzy. Later on something else happens and she is kept in the nursery or put in an incubator, or maybe Mom has difficulties and has to be taken into surgery. These circumstances intensify the original emotions produced at the birth experience. Some time later little Suzy gets separated from Mommy at the shopping mall and becomes terrified, and the security people have to find Mommy. As time goes on, Mommy and Daddy separate and then get divorced, which serves to create even more feelings of abandonment. As little Suzy gets older she may have difficulty when a parent needs to leave her alone for any length of time. Maybe she has trouble going off to school and being away from Mommy. These events add to the SSE experiences. The SSE experiences may not seem like much at the time, but they are continuing to compound the original feelings of abandonment.

As little Suzy becomes big Suzy, she gets married and moves out on her own. Initially life seems to be pretty good for Suzy; however, her abandonment issues show up as control in regard to her new husband. He becomes disillusioned, finding himself being suffocated by Suzy's jealousy. He's had it with her controlling him and her needing to be aware of where he is every moment. She finally suffocates him to the point where he wants out of the relationship. Suzy responds with panic attacks or some sort of emotional breakdown. This incident is what we refer to as the SPE, or Symptom Producing Event. This is the point where people will show up in the therapist's office.

The SPE occurs when a person's normal coping strategies break down and they are now face-to-face with their issue. Avoidance is probably the most common coping strategy that people use. For someone like Suzy, she may have avoided situations that would bring up feelings of abandonment—like overnight stays with friends, or summer camp, or other similar activities that would take her away from Mommy and familiar surroundings. As Suzy got older she may have picked a college close to home, or created co-dependencies with others to help her feel secure. And that cell phone at hand kept Mom and others as close as a speed dial away.

Any incidents of a similar nature that occur after the SPE are referred to as SIEs, or Symptom Intensifying Events. These SIEs are similar to SSEs; however, they follow the SPE. If Suzy fails to get help, her life at this point could take a turn for the worse. She could end up becoming so frozen by her fears that she may be unable to function at any sort of acceptable level.

I like to think of this whole process as a row of dominoes. As shown in Figure 5, the ISE is the first domino and it is followed by a lot of other dominoes that are SSEs. Somewhere down that row of dominoes is the SPE, followed by a number of dominoes that are SIEs.

Some therapists will simply begin regressing their client back. They may get them back to one of the SSEs and find that's as far as they can get their client to go. Often I've heard them say things like, "This is as far as the subconscious mind is willing to go at this time and the client will need to come back next week." Or they will say that the client is resistant and won't be able to continue on, or (due to the resistance) it will take a lot of work to move them ahead.

There is also a belief that no matter how far back (down the row of dominos) you get, everything that occurred after is resolved. There seems to be some truth to that, as if all the dominoes after that point just topple over (as is shown in Figure 5), but you can't count on it. Sometimes a client will actually experience relief by getting partially down that row of dominoes. (I know because I've done it.)

Dave Elman, author of the book *Hypnotherapy,* was one of the greatest hypnotists of all time. Yet, after reading his transcripts, I discovered that much of the regression he did never got to the ISE. Elman certainly had a good deal of success though. Some of that, I believe, had to do with the period of time during which Elman practiced and the fact that it was *Dave Elman* doing the hypnosis. I also believe that, at times, people walk into the office and they are just ready to be over their issue. The mind is a powerful thing and when it's ready to make a change, the hypnotist could read to the client from the phone directory and that would resolve their issue. That may be the case, but do keep in mind that getting to the ISE is the most *sure* way to get to the cause and resolve the client's issue (see Figure 6).

I will use an example of a woman who came to see me from out of state. She had recently developed a strong fear of flying (a very common issue), which had never been a problem before. When I began regressing her, she went back to a very recent flight going to Las Vegas. She and her boyfriend were traveling with some of their

Figure 5

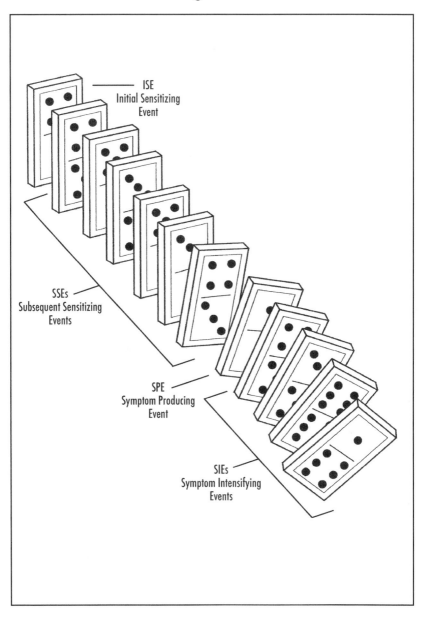

Figure 6

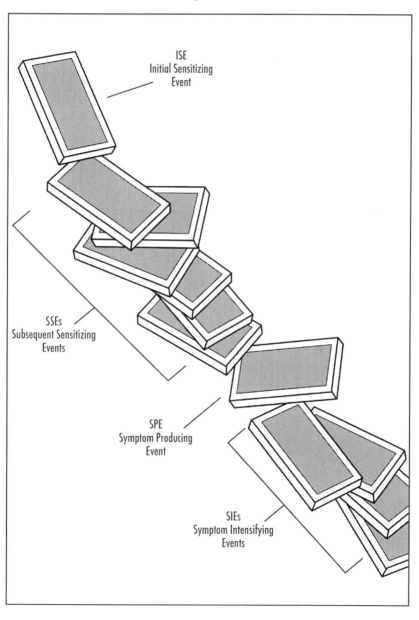

ISE
Initial Sensitizing
Event

SSEs
Subsequent Sensitizing
Events

SPE
Symptom Producing
Event

SIEs
Symptom Intensifying
Events

friends for an extended weekend of partying, which would seem like a fun thing. She began emoting very strongly and I inquired as to the nature of these feelings. It seems she had recently become pregnant and her boyfriend had convinced her to get an abortion, and now she was flying to Vegas and stewing in her grief. From this point on, every time she got on a plane it triggered these same feelings of grief. We did a Gestalt piece (I'll explain in greater detail later on) around the unborn child. She was immediately relieved of her emotional discomfort and was able to fly again in total comfort. In this example, I did not regress this person to an ISE and there is still a strong likelihood that those emotions she was feeling on the plane may have had a much earlier connection. In her case, however, doing the Gestalt piece was enough to break the connection that she had created with her feelings and flying.

Sometimes it seems as though an ISE has occurred much later in life. It appears to me that there are times when a person's paradigms become so significantly shattered that an ISE is created. I have only noticed this in a few individuals. I believe that, as youngsters, it is necessary for us to experience a certain amount of adversity. Certainly we want to avoid abuse towards children; however, some adversity early in life helps to teach us that we *can* get through difficulties and move ahead with our lives. It helps that parents or other support people are there to help make these incidents easier to deal with.

It has been my experience that there are times when a person has been raised in a very sheltered environment. It could be that it's a very "Leave It to Beaver" type of situation, or it could be due to cultural circumstances, such as being brought up in a region where there is little contact with the rest of the world. An individual in this type of situation develops a paradigm that this is the way life is and nothing ever happens to challenge their paradigm. Later in life a situation like war occurs, which is totally inconsistent with their paradigms of how the world should work. Their critical factor is bypassed and an ISE occurs late in life, or at least there is the appearance of an ISE. Transformational Replay, as described in this book, will benefit this person as well.

With some rare exceptions, resistance typically occurs due to lack of ability on the part of the therapist. Dave Elman said that the only reason a client would demonstrate resistance is due to fear. This is true. He also said it is the job of the hypnotist to alleviate that fear. Right again. When we are dealing with certain issues, and especially when we are doing regression, it may be impossible to eliminate fear completely. If a therapist uses the methods I present in this text, they should be able to achieve a successful regression to the ISE without getting stuck halfway to their goal.

A therapist came to me and told me that regression therapy does not work. When I asked her why, she said it was because each time she regressed her client she got a different ISE. Even if you are not a therapist you can probably understand that she has never gotten her client to the ISE. She is simply regressing them, getting to an SSE, and assuming that the SSE is the ISE. Through the methods described in this book, a therapist will be able to more effectively get the client to the ISE and determine that it *is* the ISE.

7

Gestalt Therapy and Hypnotherapy

Gestalt therapy is a type of therapy that was the work of Fritz Perls. My wife, Lynsi, and I studied Gestalt therapy at the Gestalt Institute of the Rockies. Part of the reason that we sought out training in this therapy was because we were already using Gestalt methods in our hypnotherapy (which is common practice) and we wanted to know more about it. The term *Gestalt* means "the whole." Gestalt is a very imaginative kind of process and fits in well with the hypnotic process. In fact, many times the Gestalt therapist is working in hypnosis and is probably unaware of it. I have been witness to many Gestalt sessions and it is apparent to me that many of the clients have achieved a hypnotic trance during their process.

I'm not going to attempt to do a Gestalt training in these pages; however, there are some applications of this work that therapists need to be aware of. Probably the most widely known and used part of Gestalt is the "Two Chair" method. Let's say you have an issue with your father. With the Two Chair technique you would sit in one chair and imagine that your father is sitting in the other chair. The session might go something like this:

Therapist: (*Motioning to opposite chair*) Now, what do you need to say to your father?

Client: (*Sounding kind of timid*) You SOB.

Therapist: That's right; say it again only louder.

Client: You SOB! You ran off and left me and Mom and little Sis to struggle for ourselves. We never knew where our next meal was coming from. We wore old hand-me-downs and the kids at school made fun of us. You left Mom an emotional wreck and she's never been the same. (*The client emotes.*)

Therapist: How does that make you feel?

Client: I'm totally pissed!

Therapist: All right, Suzy, now sit in the other chair and become your father. Now, what does Father need to say to Suzy?

Client: (*As her father*) I never meant to hurt you. Your mother was drinking and having an affair; she never wanted to be with me. Your mother thought my family had money so she tricked me into getting her pregnant. I tried to stick it out for you kids, but I was losing my mind. I started drinking and seeing someone else as well.

Therapist: All right, now sit back in this chair and become Suzy again. How do you need to respond to your father?

Client: I hate you, you SOB! I just want to beat the shit out of you. (*The therapist gives the client a rubber bat and places a pillow on the opposite chair.*)

Therapist: All right, Suzy, take this bat show him how you feel.

Client: Take this you SOB! (*Client hits the pillow with the bat while screaming.*) I hate you! I hate you!

Therapist: (*With lots of enthusiasm in the voice*) That's right, tell that SOB how you feel!

Client: (*Screaming*) You worthless SOB, I hate you! You never came to see us. You never even sent a card at Christmas time! You never wanted me. I hate you, I hate you, you worthless SOB! (*This catharsis continues until the client drops in a heap.*)

Therapist: (*After assisting client back to her chair*) That's right, Suzy, now sit back in this other chair and become your father. What does your father say to you?

Client: (*As her father*) I'm sorry, I'm sorry. You're right, I am a worthless SOB. I've always felt that way since I was a little kid. When I married your mom, I was in love with her, but she was just using me. She belittled me and cheated on me and I just felt worse and worse. When I left, I was drinking and lost my job. I wanted to send you money, but I could barely feed myself. At least your mom was getting some welfare and that was more than I had. I wrote you letters and sent you cards, but they were always returned by your mother. Eventually she had moved you guys around so many times that I could no longer find you. I would lay awake nights on end worrying about you. Yes, you're right, I am a worthless SOB, but a worthless SOB that has always loved you very much. (*Client breaks down sobbing once again.*)

Therapist: Now move back to this other chair and become Suzy once again. What do you need to say to Father now?

Client: (*Suzy begins to kneel at her father's chair.*) I love you too, Daddy.

Therapist: (*Handing a pillow to Suzy*) That's right, Suzy, what else?

Client: (*While hugging the pillow tightly*) I love you too, Daddy, and I forgive you. I'm sorry for the bad things that I said about you. Somehow I knew it couldn't be entirely your fault. That witch of a mother was always telling us what a loser you were, but it's easy to see now that she was the bigger problem. I will always love you, Daddy, and I want us to spend a lot more time together. We've missed out on way too much.

Therapist: Now, become Daddy.

Client: (*As the father*) You're right, Suzy, I love you forever and we are going to make up for lost time together. I have a great new career now and a good home. We can spend lots of time together. You're such a beautiful and smart young woman; I want to be there for you from here on.

Therapist: How does that make you feel?

Client: I feel wonderful. I feel like a huge weight has been lifted from me. I feel free and hopeful. At last I feel wanted.

This is an example of how a Gestalt session might go. The session would not be limited to the two chairs described here. If there were more players in the scenario that needed to be addressed, we could create that opportunity. Sometimes a large number of pillows and pieces of furniture might represent other players in this life drama. Mom and little sis could have easily been brought into this scene.

Some therapists believe that emoting and catharsis is the goal of the Gestalt session, but that is not the case. As Gestalt therapists, we are simply assisting the client with whatever they have come in with. In the previous example, the therapist did help the client to get in touch with her anger. When Suzy first referred to her father as an SOB, she was obviously downplaying the underlying feelings of anger. The therapist only assisted her in getting real about those emotions; he did not try to create the anger for her. We support the emotions and catharsis in Gestalt therapy as well as in hypnotherapy.

Whether or not the client abreacts should not be the therapist's goal. Facilitating the client in their emotional moment is our duty. Facilitation does not mean that we try to comfort them or make them feel better; it's about letting them have their experience in a controlled environment. Therapists who are quick to take a client out of these emotional experiences either don't understand the process well, or may be uncomfortable with their own emotions. (And that sounds like the *therapist* needs a session!)

Often a great sense of relief comes after that entire pillow beating and yelling and screaming. This can be an important part of the healing process; however, it is not the goal of the session. Some therapists do session after session of beating up pillows and yelling and screaming, over and over again. How long is this to go on? Is the client healing? Anger is an emotion that evokes action, and physical action is a good way to dispel the anger. However, if we continue beating up Mother or whoever, session after session, aren't we eventually just reinforcing the rage and anger?

I encourage my clients to get involved in vigorous exercise (for many issues). Exercise helps us to feel better about ourselves. People with anger issues can work that off in the gym rather than on their family members. The more vigorous and demanding the exercise is, the better, when dealing with anger (going to total exhaustion at times can be good). Use common sense when it comes to exercise: Get a physical, get a trainer, and be smart about it.

Remember that if the therapist insists that the session culminates in catharsis, then the therapist has his or her own agenda. The agenda for the session must be about the client's issues and not about how the therapist wants the outcome to happen.

The process of Gestalt therapy translates easily into the hypnotic process. In fact, it works much better in a hypnotic session. With hypnotherapy the Gestalt takes place with the client already in a trance state and we have the advantage of trance logic working in our favor. In hypnosis there is no need to set up chairs or pillows; the subconscious mind will take care of all of that for us. Once the client is in the desired trance state, it can be as easy as saying something like:

Therapist: Experience your father in front of you. What do you need to say to your father? (*This wording needs to be given in a very directive manner and without hesitation. If the therapist is not direct or hesitates at this point, the client may start to engage the conscious mind and the momentum can be lost. If the therapist uses permissive language like, "You can see your father standing in front of you now if you're ready," the same problem may arise. The skill of the therapist keeps this process moving and helps to bring a rapid resolution to the issue.*)

Client: Why did you leave us, you SOB?

After this the client may respond as their father, or the therapist simply says, "What is your father's response?" Or, "How does your father respond?"

Client: He says he's never done anything wrong and it was my entire fault.

Sometimes the response may be something like, "He won't say anything; he just stands there with that smug look on his face." In this case the therapist needs to take a slightly different tack:

Therapist: All right, Suzy, who can take control with him? Who can we bring in here that can make that SOB respond?

Client: Well, Granny always knew how to make him pay attention and mind.

Therapist: Bring Granny into the middle of this scene. What does Granny need to say to your father to make him understand?

Client: Granny grabs him by the ear and shoves a bar of soap into his mouth. He's crying and pleading for mercy. She tells him he needs to fess up and come clean.

Therapist: What's happening now?

Client: He says, please, please, I'm sorry, I know what I did was wrong. I promise I'll do whatever I can to make it up.

Therapist: How does that make you feel?

Client: I feel a lot better, but that SOB needs to pay for what he's done.

Therapist: What would be an appropriate punishment for Father?

Client: That lazy SOB needs to be put to work digging ditches and all of his earnings should go to all of the kids he has neglected.

If the client fails to come up with a solution readily on their own—and it is best if they come up with their own solution—then I may give some suggestions like: "Maybe you could lock him up in a cell filled with movie projectors that are playing his lies and perpetrations over and over." The client is the only one with the key and he or she can let the perpetrator out whenever they see fit. This helps to put the client in control.

Therapist: That's right, how does that make you feel?

Client: I feel much more in control.

Therapist: What about Granny?

Client: Granny's great! She says she has plenty of soap and those big bullies don't scare her none. She says whenever I need her just holler. (*This will help to build support for the client.*)

It's best when the client creates the changes in the inner world themselves. That way they are putting themselves in charge of their own process. Even if the therapist knows exactly what the client may need, it's more empowering when the client finds it for him- or herself so they can own the process.

This particular scenario could have played out in many different ways. The client may have decided to take matters into his or her own hands and beat the crap out of Father. I keep a plastic bat behind the recliner in my office and big pillows handy. A good hypnotherapist is not there to lead the client's session. If the therapist had suggested bringing in the police, that might have worked; but the client may not have owned it, or may have even resented the therapist meddling in their session. The therapist may have never considered Granny for the job, but Granny knew Father when he was young and probably put the fear of God into him then. Therefore, she was a good choice.

The Gestalt can be done with anyone, whether alive or dead, even if we've never met the person. Someone could have issues with an absent parent (they may have become estranged early on, or have been adopted) and would like some resolution. Often I have connected clients with an aborted child to help relieve guilt and grief around that issue. Connecting someone with that aborted child has been a most positive session experience, and not just for the mothers. Recall the incident of the young woman flying to Las Vegas: Connecting her with that aborted child is what made all the difference for her.

One of the reasons that Gestalt works so well in hypnosis is due to *Trance Logic.* Trance logic allows the mind to go places that wouldn't make sense in the conscious, waking state. If I were talking to someone out on the street and said, "See that big purple buffalo standing in front of you," that person would probably think I was crazy. But in trance, the subconscious mind will go right there without hesitation. The Gestalt is often part of the Transformational Replay, but it is also effective on its own.

8

Anchors and Triggers

I am including anchors and triggers here, because they play a significant enough role in the Transformational Replay process that they need to be addressed. When I teach the use of anchors and triggers to my students, I like to demonstrate how they can be used. Usually I will ask for a volunteer. I have the volunteer stand with me in front of the class. Then I will ask the volunteer to close their eyes and recall an unpleasant incident from their past. When they have brought that incident up, they let me know. I ask them to become aware of sensations in the body that they are noticing until they have fully experienced the sensations.

I then ask them to recall another event, only a much more pleasant event, like Christmas morning, finding that new bicycle under the tree, or something similar that feels good. When the volunteer is fully in that moment, I ask them to notice the good sensations associated with this new scene. I ask them to become aware of how and where they experience these sensations in their body. As they do this, I place my hand on their shoulder. When I remove my hand, I ask them to recall another positive experience—maybe a vacation or falling in love. Once they are in that place in their mind they let me know and I ask them again to notice those feelings in their body and how it feels, as I place my hand on their shoulder. Then I ask them to go to a third pleasant experience similar to the first two and, once again, as they are becoming involved in the enjoyable feelings, I place my hand on their shoulder (keeping it there for a while in each instance).

I then ask them to bring up the image of that first uncomfortable incident once again. When they let me know that they have this incident clearly in their mind, I place my hand on their shoulder and, amazingly, they will report that the emotions connected with that first experience have diminished considerably.

What just happened? Often the class members don't have a clue as to what just happened. Each time the student accessed a positive emotional image I placed my hand on their shoulder—something I did *not* do with the original uncomfortable image. My hand on the student's shoulder became associated with the feelings of each enjoyable memory. Creating that association is what we call *anchoring*. So now the good feelings and the touch on the shoulder have a positive association. When I had the student recall the uncomfortable memory the final time, I placed my hand on the shoulder. This gesture was now associated with positive feelings, causing the uncomfortable feelings to be diminished. This is a hypnosis tool commonly associated with Neurolinguistic Programming (NLP).

Anchors and triggers are nothing new—they've been around all along. Another example I use with my class is to ask a student to pretend to be Mrs. Instructor. I pretend to be coming home and handing her a dozen roses. Then I turn to the class and I ask what is happening here? Invariably they respond with, "What have you done wrong?" Why? Because, sad to say, this is the association we have managed to create with bringing flowers home to our wives. When something is going wrong with a couple, that's when the guy brings home flowers. He's trying to do the right thing and to make things better, but the problem is that flowers have been anchored to bad situations. If the only time that flowers are brought home is to fix things that have gone wrong, then every time flowers show up it means something bad is happening. Just ask Danny Bonaduce.

Guys, pay attention! If you want flowers to work for you, you have to bring her flowers (and often!) when things are going great. That way you are anchoring the flowers to good feelings. Later if there is a problem, the flowers might actually help change things (trigger good feelings), rather than become a potential weapon against you.

Have you ever been aware of a situation where someone is feeling down and their special person tries to hug them to make things better, only to get pushed away and met with resistance? Again, someone cares and wants to make things better; however, if we only hug and comfort each other when there is something out of sorts, then we're just anchoring the hugs with uncomfortable feelings. We need to hug and comfort each other more often (when things are going great), so that we create a positive anchor and the hugs will actually have a positive affect.

Maybe you've been driving down the road listening to the radio and a certain song comes on, and suddenly you've just been transported back to that high school dance when you asked Mary Lou to go steady. I remember driving through the country with my father as the smell of manure became strong and Dad responded with "oooooh, yuck, the farm," and I responded with "aaaaah, the farm." We had two totally different responses to the same trigger. I had a girlfriend once named Sandy, whose middle name was Sue. I referred to her one day as Sandra Sue and she turned and snarled at me. I don't know who referred to her as Sandra Sue in the past, but it was definitely anchored with not-so-good feelings.

Mothers have used anchors and triggers since the beginning of time. When Mom gave you *that look,* you knew she meant business and it was time to straighten up. *That look* might be accompanied by her arms crossed in front of her body, with maybe some toe tapping or a pointing finger. The reason *that look* (the trigger) has been so effective is because at some point it was anchored with some serious punishment and now *that look* is all it takes to get the results that Mom desires.

I've had people ask me if I could hypnotize their dog to do what they want it to do. When training our dogs, we already use hypnosis in the form of anchors and triggers. When Ole Blue is lying down with us watching TV and he's very relaxed, you might be scratching him on his favorite spot behind his ears. What you have done is unknowingly create an anchor and trigger. He now associates being scratched behind his ears with the feelings of being very relaxed. Later, someone comes to the door and Ole Blue starts howling and getting upset. When you start scratching Ole Blue behind the ears (the trigger), it causes him to feel the relaxed sensations that are associated with the scratching. We do the same thing when we're training a dog. When the dog does something right, it's given a reward like a doggy treat or a pat on the head.

If any of this *anchors and triggers* business sounds to you like Pavlovian response or conditioned response, you are correct. Like many great discoveries, conditioned response was accidental. Pavlov was studying saliva production in dogs when he found that certain things (triggers) would stimulate more saliva production. Better for Pavlov to be known for conditioned response than dog saliva.

Hypnotists take advantage of anchors and triggers in a variety of ways. Stage hypnotists create anchors in their subjects to deepen their trance or to trigger some other response. Stage hypnotists often use a hand on a participant's shoulder or a sound to anchor sensations of relaxation. Then whenever the hypnotist wants to deepen someone, all he needs to do is place his hand on his or her shoulder or make a certain sound and the participant sinks deeper into relaxation (not unlike the way I used my hand on my student's shoulder to anchor the good feelings).

During the Transformational Replay process we use anchors (which are usually kinesthetic anchors, physical anchors like the touch on the shoulder) to anchor positive feelings that the client can now access on their own whenever they may desire. It's necessary to anchor only those positive feelings of the greatest significance. Later, as I describe the process in greater detail, you will have a clear understanding of how that works and why we do it in the manner that we do.

9

Dissociation and the Hypnotic Process

Dissociation can be a psychological survival method or it can be a tool that we use in the hypnotic trance. We all dissociate from time to time: Daydreaming is a form of dissociation. If we want to escape an uncomfortable (boring) moment, we might find ourselves daydreaming about some more appealing fantasy. When someone totally blocks out the memory of a past event, this is also *dissociation*. If we choose to remember things differently from how they actually occurred, or if we are in denial about something, that is also dissociation. People who have been perpetrators of horrendous abuse will often go into denial or simply choose to recall their perpetration in some other way. For a lot of people, admitting to committing those actions is so inconsistent with the paradigms they have about themselves, that the identity they have presented to the world just doesn't equate to reality. To admit to such atrocities would also mean they are admitting to being crazy, because who other than a crazy person could perform such heinous acts?

In hypnotherapy we sometimes can make use of the mind's natural ability to dissociate. For instance, if a client gets into a scene from the past that is so emotionally paralyzing that they are unable to move ahead, then we can suggest that the client dissociate. A dissociative technique may go something like: "Okay, now experience this scene as if you were watching it from a distance, or on a stage, or view it as you would view a video tape. You have the remote control and can pause it, or stop it, or slow it down, or whatever." If I was working with a Vietnam veteran viewing an uncomfortable battle scene, we could place him in a helicopter to view the scene from a safer distance.

There are many possible ways to dissociate in these kinds of situations. I tell my students that it is necessary to know these dissociative techniques, but there's rarely any need for them. Some therapists jump into dissociative methods as soon as things start to get emotional. Oftentimes the therapist is jumping into these methods because they, themselves, are not comfortable with emotions. The truth is we need the emotions that come up to create the affect bridge that will eventually take us to the ISE. The moment we start to use a dissociative technique we may lose our momentum. It is not necessary to keep a client in an uncomfortable moment indefinitely, but neither do we want to rob them of their experience by moving them along too quickly. Once we have experienced the emotions in that scene, we can then use the emotions to move the client toward the ISE (the emotions being the affect bridge).

I have had some clients who spend most of their time in a dissociative state. It's as though they are watching their entire life as if it were taking place on a stage. This way they can avoid having to deal with any emotions that might come up.

A man brought his wife to see me several years back. She was having anxiety, particularly around driving, and was not experiencing normal feelings. In hypnosis she re-experienced a time that she had previously blocked from conscious memory. She was married to a previous husband and lived in California. At that point in her life, my client had never lived outside of southern California, and so she had never seen any snow. Her husband thought it was time for her to finally experience snow, so they headed to the Redwood Forest with another couple. Her husband was driving a bit too fast in a big, old Buick. They went through a tunnel and at the end of the tunnel there was a cliff wall on one side of the road and a rock guard wall on the other. A husband and wife, along with their young son, had stopped there to look over the wall and take in the view. My client's then-husband lost control, and their large car headed into the cliff. The car glanced off the cliff and veered into the small family standing at the rock wall. The entire family was cut in half as the car smashed them against the wall. The woman and child died immediately, but the father lingered for some time, looking up at my client saying, "Why? Why?"

My client was so traumatized by the horror of this event that she could not face her own emotions around what had just happened. She began dissociating her entire life. From that point on, she went through life viewing it as if she were simply an observer watching it, and not an active participant in it. This saved her from having to deal with her own feelings and allowed her to function in her world. The problem with this strategy is that while there is the illusion of being protected from those uncomfortable emotions, there is also the loss of being involved in her own life.

In this instance, the Gestalt worked very well. While she was in trance, I had my client interact with the father as he was dying on the road. Forgiveness was attained in the process and my client was able to get in touch with her own feelings once again. The process was successful for my client. She said this was the first time since that accident that she had ever been able to cry. When her husband brought her to her next appointment, he told me that he didn't know what I had done, but his wife was a whole new woman. He said they had been taking her to different psychologists for years and had tried numerous medications and this was the only thing that had ever worked. My client now felt safe to drive and could get herself to work and anywhere else she chose.

Denial and delusion are also forms of dissociation and people can become so deluded that there is almost no truth to what they present as their reality.

So dissociation can be a tool (use it sparingly) or it can be a strategy that people use to protect themselves from uncomfortable sensations.

10

A Fear of Wrists

About eight years ago I received a phone call from a woman asking if I could help her daughter to overcome her fear of wrists. I am told that there are over two thousand named phobias. I have one list of several hundred different phobias. The DSMIV manual (the diagnostic manual used by therapists to help diagnose clients for insurance and other purposes) lists some of the major phobias, and others fall under groupings. A person could develop a phobia around anything given the right set of circumstances. When my client's mother called I knew I could help her daughter, even though I had never heard of fear of wrists before. I did, however, know how to use hypnotherapy, and I knew that my skills could be applied to whatever phobia a person might come in with.

During the intake portion of our session I discovered that my client couldn't stand anything to do with wrists. She didn't want to see them or talk about them. She wore long sweaters and blouses so as to cover her own wrists so she wouldn't have to notice them. She would not wear bracelets or watches, for that would only bring attention to her wrists. Her boyfriend had to be very careful when holding hands with her so as to not touch her wrists in any way. That very morning she had just had a manicure and everything went fine until the manicurist started to put lotion on her hands. My client became totally freaked out.

The phobia was around other people's wrists as well as her own. Even department store mannequins, whose wrists were visible, created discomfort for my client. All I had to do to bring up her fear of wrists was to say, "I'm thinking about your wrist," and she would start cringing and squirming in her chair. Along with her fear of wrists was a fear of needles and she said that the two things were strongly connected.

My client was an x-ray technician, working in a hospital in a large city on the east coast. Of course, I asked about the fact that wrists certainly must come up during her normal job. That was indeed the case, but she described ways that she had learned to get around those situations (the coping strategies that I talked about earlier). Some of her strategies included getting a colleague to perform those duties, or covering that part of the body, or just holding her breath until it was all over. Normally, injections (her fear of needles) would have been a problem; however, she worked in a state where x-ray technicians did not give injections. This was a problem now, because she was moving to a different state and was going to work in a new hospital where she would be expected to give injections to patients. This was her SPE (symptom producing event)—the point at which her usual coping strategies were no longer effective. So her mother had called me to make her appointment.

During the interview I found out that her childhood was pretty normal except for some of the incidents around her SSEs (subsequent sensitizing events). At one point she recounted what had happened when she was about four years old. She had been shopping with her maternal grandmother at a large department store when she got her sleeve caught in an escalator and her wrist was broken. This seemed like a very traumatic incident that certainly could have created her ISE (the initial sensitizing event) and I certainly thought this must be the case. (Recall that I said earlier that the ISE is not remembered—with some exceptions that I will explain later—so her recollection of the ISE could indicate cause for concern.)

I encourage checking a client's SUDs (Subsequent Units of Distress) level when doing this type of work. The SUDs scale is a system that many therapists use to determine the level of distress that their client is experiencing. This scale is simply a scale from one to ten. A one on the scale would mean that the client is experiencing no distress and a ten would mean that the distress is unbearable. While doing something to evoke my client's distress (like touching her wrist, which she would not tolerate), I'd ask, "Where are you on a scale of one to ten?" She was way at the top of the scale without me actually touching her wrist. In her case all I had to do was say "I'm looking at your wrist" or "I'm thinking about your wrists" and this would be more than enough to cause her to writhe and squeal in her chair.

The following session, working with this client's fear of wrists, is very typical of how I normally deal with a phobia. Remember that this all happens in only a single session.

After the intake and induction to a safe place (which I do to create safety for clients and to allow them to experience interaction in trance in a simple way):

Me: Tell me what you see or feel [*in the safe place*].

Client: It's a beautiful garden.

Me: Describe your surroundings.

Client: There are lots of green plants and flowers. There's a small waterfall and the little stream trickles through the garden.

Me: Notice the temperature of the air on your skin, how does that feel?

Client: It feels warm, but not too warm. It's just a little bit humid, very pleasant.

Me: Notice the sky, and tell me what kind of day it is.

Client: It's sunny with a few fluffy clouds floating around.

Me: Do you notice any sounds?

Client: The sound of the waterfall is very pleasant; there are some birds and just a slight breeze in the trees.

Me: Are there any smells?

Client: There's the smell of flowers and just clean air.

Me: That's right, now take a deep breath and breathe in these good feelings of comfort, relaxation and safety. This is your special place and it's just right for you and you can come here any time you wish—any time you wish at all—to just relax, to be creative, or to solve some problem in a positive manner. This is your special place and it's just right for you. Now, take in a deep breath and breathe in these good feelings and feel yourself going deeper. (*This helps to build a self-hypnosis resource and deepen the client.*) Now take a deep breath and feel yourself drifting back in time, back in time to a happy, carefree time, a happy carefree time where you are being very active. Perhaps you are involved in some sporting event as a youngster or some childhood game, or some other activity that causes you to use your body in a vigorous manner. It's a happy time, an active time. (*This helps to show your client that they can travel in time in a non-threatening way, which helps to eliminate resistance later.*) Tell me what's happening now.

Client: I'm riding my bicycle on the street in front of our house.

Me: How old are you?

Client: I'm five years old.

Me: What are you wearing?

Client: I'm wearing my blue shorts with a red tank top; my bicycle is silver with a banana seat.

Me: Are you alone or with someone?

Client: My big sister is here, we're racing up the hill, and we're laughing and screaming.

Me: That's right, notice how good it feels to use your young muscles, so strong, so limber, so full of energy, it feels like you can just go on and on. Take a deep breath and breathe in these good, happy, carefree feelings into every cell of your body (*a type of anchoring method*) and feel yourself sinking deeper and deeper (*this helps to deepen the client and create a transition*). In a moment I'm going to ask you to go back to a time, and you will go back to a time, you'll go back to a recent time, perhaps the most recent time, that something about wrists makes you uncomfortable. Now take a deep breath and feel yourself moving into that recent time that you experience discomfort in regard to wrists. Tell me what's happening now.

Client: I'm out shopping with my boyfriend and we're walking by some mannequins with their wrists exposed. I'm turning away and dragging my boyfriend with me. I'm trying to look away. There's another mannequin when I turn. I'm dragging my boyfriend back out the door.

Me: How does that make you feel?

Client: I'm scared. I'm shaking. (*emoting*)

Me: Where do you feel that in your body?

Client: It's in my chest, my chest feels hollow. I feel frantic, my heart is racing, and I can't breathe! (*This creates our affect bridge or somatic affect bridge; the emotions that will take us to the ISE.*)

Me: Take a deep breath and feel yourself drifting back in time, back to an earlier time when you feel these similar sensations, these frantic sensations, these hollow sensations in your chest. What's happening, what's happening now? (*This is done in a very directive manner, without hesitation, so as to keep the client in their feelings, the feelings that will take us to the ISE.*)

Client: I'm in high school. We're at the Valentines Day dance. Johnny is asking me to go steady. He's trying to put a ring on my finger and he grabs me by the wrist. I'm screaming and jerking my hand away. The ring is flying across the gym floor. (*emoting*) Johnny is hurt; I can see it in his eyes. He doesn't know what's happening. I'm so embarrassed. (*sobbing*) People are looking at us, it's awful.

Me: What are you feeling?

Client: It's that hollow sensation in my chest. I can't breathe. I'm terrified. I'm frantic.

Me: Take a deep breath, going back in time back in time to an earlier time, perhaps the very first time you feel these frantic sensations, hollow sensations, in your chest. Be there now. What's happening?

Client: I'm with Grandma and we're shopping at one of those big department stores. I love going shopping with Grandma; she always buys me some neat stuff. We're going down the escalator and I'm excited and talking with Grandma. I'm running my hand along the rail on the escalator. Oh my God (*client starts screaming and crying*), my sleeve is caught in the thing! I'm screaming! Grandma's trying to help! She's pulling on my sleeve, Grandma, Grandma! Help me! We're coming to the bottom, my arm won't come out! Oh my God! My sleeve is ripping lose. I've pulled free, but I hurt, my wrist, it hurts so bad!

Me: What else are you feeling?

Client: I feel that hollow feeling in my chest! I'm frantic! I'm scared!

Me: Are these feelings that you are familiar with or are these new, unusual feelings and sensations?

Client: They're familiar.

Me: Go back, back in time, back to the very first time you feel these feelings and sensations.

Client: I'm almost three years old. Daddy has taken me to meet my grandparents for the very first time. They are in some kind of hospital (*actually both grandparents are dying and her dad wants her to meet them before they die*), it's big and scary. Dad seems nervous too. I'm going into a room with Daddy. He takes me to a bed where an old woman is lying. She looks scary. She has a hard time talking, or moving. Daddy says to come closer so Grandma can meet you. I'm scared, I don't like this. Oh my God! She has a big needle shoved in her wrist! (*screaming and emoting*)

Me: What's happening now?

Client: I'm running down the hall screaming! I want to go home. Daddy's running after me, I'm screaming and crying! I'm terrified! I can't breathe! I feel that awful feeling in my chest!

Me: Have you ever felt these feelings and sensations prior to this time?

Client: I've never felt like this before.

Me: Now take a deep breath, and imagine this scene starting over from the beginning just like rewinding a tape, only this time imagine this scene happening over in a whole, new, healthier, better way—a way that works better for you. In fact, imagine your adult self coming into this scene and taking control of this new, better scene.

Client: Adult me is with me and Daddy and she's holding me and telling me we are going to meet Grandma. She helps to make Daddy feel better too. She knows how to make me feel safer. She holds me and makes me feel safe. She tells me that Grandma has been feeling badly, but she loves me very much and wants to meet me. We go in the room and I can see Grandma, she's all covered up. She's really skinny, but she's talking to me very pleasantly. She asks if I remember talking to her on the phone. She reaches out and touches my face and tells me how pretty I am. She takes a gold band from her finger and says this is to be mine. She says her grandma gave it to her a long, long time ago.

Me: How does that make you feel?

Client: It feels really good; adult me makes me feel safe, and Grandma gave me this neat ring.

Me: Where do you feel these new, good feelings in your body?

Client: I feel them in my chest.

Me: That's right. Now just place your hand on your chest where you notice these new, good, safe feelings. (*The client places her hand on her chest.*) Now notice these new, good, safe feelings in your chest. Feel these new, good, safe feelings building right there beneath your hand. Notice how good that feels. Any time you wish to feel these new, good, safe feelings all you have to do is touch your chest in this very manner and feel these good, safe feelings building right there beneath your hand. (*This creates the anchor that the client can now trigger on her own when she desires.*) Now take a deep breath and breathe these new, safe feelings deep into every cell of your body. (*This helps to further anchor the new feelings.*)

Me: Now let's go back to the time when you were shopping at the big department store with your maternal grandma and there was the escalator incident. Imagine this scene happening over in a whole, new, healthier way, a way that works better for you, and tell me what's happening.

Client: I'm with Grandma and we've been shopping. We have packages that we're carrying as we get on the escalator. I start running my hands on the railing and Grandma says that's not a good idea. We need to be careful when riding on the escalator.

Me: How does that make you feel?

Client: It feels good just going shopping with Grandma.

Me: Now go back to the time when you're at the Valentine's Day dance and Johnny is asking you to go steady. Imagine this scene happening over in a whole, new, healthier way, a way that works better for you and tell me what's happening.

Client: I'm at the dance and I'm excited to be with Johnny. We've been kind of seeing each other and I think he's really cute. I can tell he's kind of nervous as he shows me a ring and he's asking me if I will go steady with him. I'm stunned and smiling, but nothing is coming out of my mouth as he slips the ring on my finger. I smile and tell him thank you as I put my arms around his neck and give him a big kiss. Lots of other kids are watching, but we don't even notice them.

Me: How does that make you feel?

Client: I feel amazing.

Me: Now take a deep breath and breathe these good feelings deep into every cell of your body. Now allow yourself to go back to that recent time when you're at the department store with your boyfriend and imagine this scene happening over in a whole, new, healthier way, a way that works better for you. Tell me what's happening.

Client: I'm shopping with my boyfriend. We're at the perfume counter and I'm trying on different samples and he's sniffing each one. We're laughing and being silly. It feels great.

Me: Now take a deep breath and breathe in these good feelings and sensations deep into every cell of your body. Now allow yourself to drift ahead in time. Perhaps to a time that would have been a challenge for you in the past and tell me what's happening now.

Client: I'm at my new job in Chicago. I'm taking x-rays of a guy's wrist. He's a construction worker and he got his arm caught while moving a load of lumber. I'm carefully moving his arm around to get it just right for the x-ray machine. He's gotten a pretty nasty cut that has been stitched and I already gave him a tetanus shot.

Me: How does that make you feel?

Client: I feel confident. It feels great!

Me: That's right. Now take a deep breath and breathe these good feelings deep into every cell of your body. Now take a deep breath and imagine yourself moving into the future once again. You're back home with your boyfriend and you're shopping at the department store. You haven't told him that you've been to see me yet. You start going up to all of the mannequins and turning their hands around backwards. (*Client laughs.*) Your boyfriend is looking at you like you're crazy, but you're just laughing and playing. (*The client laughs some more.*) Now take a deep breath and breathe these good feelings deep into every cell of your body. You may allow yourself to sink as deeply as you desire now, for I will not be asking any more questions. You can sink deeper down, as all of these new, good feelings and sensations take complete and thorough effect upon you. Every day now in every way you're moving ahead in a whole, new, positive manner. You may remember any of this you wish to remember. You may return any time you wish to return and I encourage you to return to your special place and use it for any purpose that serves you in a positive manner. In a moment I'm going to count from one to five. When I reach the count of five your eyes will be open you will be wide awake feeling better than before. (*I then count the client up.*)

Once the client has emerged from trance, I check in and ask how she is doing. Then I ask her to place her hand on her chest in that same manner as she did a moment ago in trance. As she places her hand on her chest I ask her to notice those good safe feelings building right there beneath her hand. "Do you feel those good safe feelings there beneath your hand?"

Client: Yes, yes I do.

Me: And just know that anytime you wish to feel these good feelings all you have to do is place your hand on your chest just in this very manner.

At this time I could ask the client what her SUDs level is now. Sometimes I would, but this time I just reach over and grab her arm by the wrist. I flopped her arm all around, holding her by the wrist. She was completely comfortable with that, so there was no need to even ask what her SUDs level is.

The client's mother had been sitting out in the waiting room during the session. I went out to the waiting room and told her mom to come into my office. I told her to go to her daughter and grab her by the wrist. Her mother said there was no way she could do that. I told her no, no, that it was okay; that she was fine now. When her mother came into my office she still wouldn't believe me, and she told her daughter that I said she should grab her by the wrist. Her daughter then offered her wrist out to her. Mom was more amazed than my client that she could grab her by the wrist and manipulate her arm.

This may seem like a fairly small thing, having a fear of wrists. But how much had this person's life been affected by her fears? Though she seemed to function normally, it's easy to see that her professional life was at risk, which created the SPE. Her romantic life was affected. It probably affected her normal nurturing process since her own mother had to be careful how she touched her. Then there were all of the things that may have gone on that we weren't aware of. Her whole life was changed and it happened in just one session. I've tried lots of other methods and some do work occasionally, but rarely in just one session. Other methods only help someone cope with their issue, but they may still have the issue.

Let's take a look at our row of dominoes as it relates to my client with the fear of wrists. (See Figure 7.)

Phobia is a very common issue that responds well to the Transformational Replay process. When working with phobias it's important to test your client with the SUDs level I described previously. In addition, I keep lots of props in my office to help stimulate a person's fears. I keep lots of creepy, crawly things like rubber snakes, spiders, worms and bugs. I like to confront my client with these objects (whichever one is applicable to their particular phobia) to see what their response is like. After the session I present the client with the same object that stimulated their fears prior to the session. This accomplishes two things. It helps us to be certain that the therapy we just performed was successful and it proves to the client that the fear is gone.

When working with fear of heights I like to take clients to the building stairwell or roof access. Sometimes just looking out the window of a building is enough to trigger the client's fears. If no tall buildings are handy you may be able to keep a ladder around; sometimes it doesn't take much of a ladder to trigger the clients fears. It's not always possible to have the proper props. In this case the therapist can suggest that the client imagine themselves confronted with their particular trigger. Then check their SUDs level.

I had a young man who came to me for fear of heights. He was in training to become a firefighter. Part of his training program required him to climb some very tall ladders and this was a big problem for him. He didn't think that I could get rid of his fear, but he

Figure 7
Dominoes for the Young Woman
with the Wrist Phobia

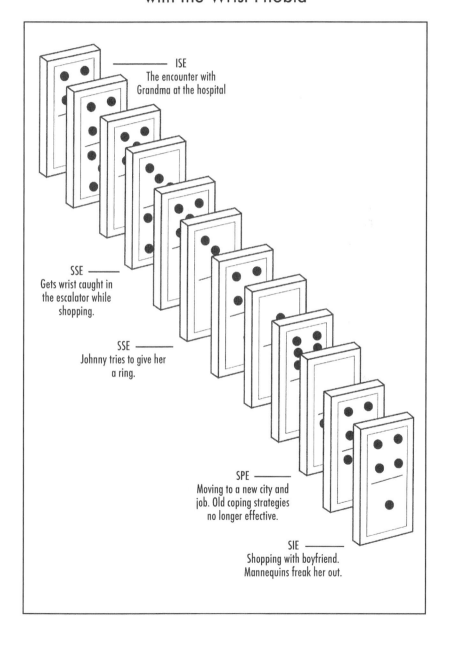

ISE
The encounter with
Grandma at the hospital

SSE
Gets wrist caught in
the escalator while
shopping.

SSE
Johnny tries to give her
a ring.

SPE
Moving to a new city and
job. Old coping strategies
no longer effective.

SIE
Shopping with boyfriend.
Mannequins freak her out.

had hopes that I could make it easier for him. Next door to my office was a much larger office building. This other office building had a parking garage underneath that went up three floors. This parking garage was open to the outdoors. I took my client to the third floor parking level. He had trouble looking out from the parking area. When I climbed up on the railing it totally freaked him out. After our session we went back to the parking garage and this time *he* climbed up on the railing.

I worked with a woman on some issues around stress and weight. She responded well to the work we were doing, and mentioned to me that she also had a fear of heights and someday would probably come back to see me. Not long after, she called and set an appointment. Her sons were coming to visit from out of state and she and her husband would be showing them around Colorado. Her fear of heights prevented her from going on mountain roads and she could no longer avoid these (one of her coping strategies) if she was going to spend time with her sons (the SPE).

I shared an office with a chiropractor in a local bank building at that time. Near the entrance to the bank building was a glassed-in area that overlooked offices in a garden level floor below. I asked my client if upon entering the building she had ever noticed that glassed-in area. She said that she had noticed, but avoided getting anywhere near it. I asked her what was down there. She said she didn't know and didn't want to know. I took her down the hallway to the glassed-in area. She was extremely upset. While I held on to the wall and she held on to my other hand she edged closer to the glass. She was trembling and screaming and was never able to see what was on that lower level. I also took her to the upper floor of the building and had her look down the stairwell. If you look down a flight of stairs between the stairs it can cause a good sensation of heights. This experiment put her at the top of her SUDs level.

We went back to my office and did her Transformational Replay session. When her session was over, she looked at me and said; "So, you think that's going to cure my fear of heights?" I took her by the hand and said, "Let's find out." She responded with, "You're not going to take me back to that hall, are you?" I said, "Of course I am." She said, "You don't think I'm going to look through that glass do you?" I said, "Yes, I do."

When we got down the hall she walked right up to the glass and put her face against the glass and said; "I can't believe I'm doing this! I can't believe I'm doing this!" She stood there in amazement repeating that same statement several times. We went back to my office and sat down. She said, "That was amazing. Do you think that will work for the stairs as well?" I said, "Let's go see." We went back to the top of the stairwell and she stood there looking down through the stairwell saying, "I can't believe I'm doing this! I can't believe I'm doing this!"

Showing the client that the work we've just done has been successful tends to keep it successful. The mind tends to expect that whatever has happened before is what will happen again. If, previously, we had a good experience in a situation, then that's what the mind expects will happen again.

Let's say someone is a little uncomfortable flying on airplanes, but it's never really been a big deal. Then on a flight there is some horrible turbulence that seems to be relentless. Maybe other people around them are displaying a lot of fear, which only works to exacerbate any fear that our person already has. Maybe this person is sure they are going to die and all sorts of horrible thoughts go through their mind. The next time this person gets on a plane, there may or may not be any problems with turbulence, but the mind is expecting that what has happened before is what is going to happen again. So our person is all uptight and can't relax. Any little bump in the plane ride just makes matters worse. If there's another episode with major turbulence our person may be taking a rental car back home.

Fear of flying is a very common phobia that I work with. Since 9/11, the stress level in airports has increased anxiety for even the most seasoned travelers. As many times as I have worked with clients who've come in for fear of flying, it's never been about flying. Flying is only triggering the feelings of some earlier ISE. Fear of flying usually relates to something else, such as claustrophobia, fear of heights, being out of control, or other anxiety issues. If you're a hypnothera-pist who has tried to get someone through their fear of flying by regressing them to flying experiences and did not succeed, it's because the flying experiences are not the ISE. The emotions that the flying triggers (the affect bridge) will take us to the ISE. With the Transformational Replay process we stay focused on the feelings—not the circumstances—that are associated with the issue. That will create a direct route to the ISE.

It is said that fear is learned and there is truth to that. However, we are also born with fear. The fears that we are born with can vary from individual to individual. Three fears are universal no matter what culture we grow up in. Those are fear of heights, fear of snakes, and fear of loud sounds. Even Eskimos are born with a fear of snakes and there are no snakes in their world. Why is this? Most likely these fears are a genetic response. Probably, in our genetic past, there were more poisonous snakes in our world and it behooved us to have a good respect for snakes. I grew up with snakes as pets and I'm very used to handling them and being around them. However, there have been times when I have been working in the garden and caught a glimpse of a snake out the corner of my eye and it would give me a start. I talked to a guy who worked in a reptile garden and he said the same thing. Even though snakes surrounded him all day, catching a glimpse of one would sometimes cause a startle response.

Fear of heights is probably more obvious because it's likely that in our genetic past we spent more time in trees and high places. Hav-ing a good, built-in respect for falling would be a good thing. Those that didn't have that particular genetic encoding probably didn't live to pass their genes to future generations.

Fear of loud sounds is likely to have a similar origin. In our genetic past the sound of a branch snapping could mean danger is upon us, and an immediate fight or flight response would be neces-sary. If you've ever been near a little baby when someone made a loud clap, you've seen how the baby will take off crying. What mother hasn't used a clap to get the attention of her children? In our culture, we have become desensitized to loud sounds because they are so prevalent.

It is normal to have some fears. Fear is a signal that we should be at least cautious. Having respect for high places is a good thing; however, when that fear becomes so intense that we can't stand next to a curb, or take the stairs, then it becomes a phobia. Some phobias are caused by indirect experience. Fear of snakes is common. I've had several experiences working with clients on this issue. After regressing my client to the ISE, the story goes something like this: "I'm very little. I'm crawling in the grass in the backyard. It's a hot summer day. My mommy is nearby hanging the laundry out to dry. All of sudden Mommy begins screaming. The laundry basket is flying across the lawn and laundry is flying all over the place. Mommy is jumping up and down yelling and screaming and crying. Her body is trembling with fear. She's pointing and screaming hysterically, yelling, 'Snake! Snake!' I can see the garter snake slithering across the lawn. I'm crying and screaming! I'm reaching out to Mommy, but she's too hysterical to help me. The old man who lives next door comes rushing over to see what the excitement is about. He picks up a rake and kills the snake. My heart is racing. I want my Mommy. The old man takes us in the house and gets us calmed down. He makes some tea for Mommy and picks up the laundry and hangs it while Mommy and I watch through the screen door."

This is what I call catching a phobia. The little baby crawling around on the grass may have experienced very little anxiety to the garter snake. It was Mommy's response to the snake that created the fear in the child. From the child's point of view, this little creature in the grass has some amazing powers. After all, the child's whole world just came crashing down. The one person in its world that was its protector and source of caring is now a total psycho. In the child's mind this little snake has some amazing powers and needs to be feared.

Early in my marriage to Lynsi, I was working in the garden with our youngest child, Dylan, who was five years old at the time. Lynsi was in the bedroom getting dressed when Dylan went in to tell her about working in the garden. All of sudden there was such screaming going on that I thought there had been some horrible accident. I raced into the bedroom where Lynsi was screaming hysterically, jumping up and down, pointing and yelling, "Spider! Spider!" As I plucked it from Dylan's shoulder, I said, "It's just a daddy-long-legs." Lynsi said, "Yeah, but I hate spiders." And I said, "Congratulations, now Dylan does too." It has been true; I've had to help rid him of that fear of spiders that he inherited from his mother in that moment of turmoil. I should mention that in both of these examples (the garter snake and the daddy-long-legs), Mom went out of control and created a strong emotional memory (a trauma perhaps) that became part of the young person's critical factor. In both cases, we know that daddy-long-legs and garter snakes are harmless, but the feelings associated are not so harmless. Remember the part about anchors and triggers? Isn't that what is happening here? Only this time very uncomfortable feelings are connected with the trigger (snakes and spiders).

Fear is a normal thing, even useful. Fear tells us to be cautious. It may even mean stop, run, or retreat, but that's not the only possibility. If we continually avoid our fears, they become increasingly large, until we become immobilized. If I had allowed my fear to stop me as I moved up the hill toward that crucifixion, my story would have played out much differently. The old adage of "when you get thrown from the horse, get right back on" is a good one. If we avoid getting on that horse, the horse just gets larger and larger until we can't get close to the horse.

Every year I go on a rafting trip down a portion of the upper Colorado River. I'm very familiar with the river and act as a guide. The group I float down the river with is made up mostly of yogis. Some are monks from India and Europe and other parts of the world. It's a group of men, and sometimes young boys, who go along with us.

One year there was a fellow who brought his two sons along. After a day or two on the river I noticed that the boat with the father and his two sons would stop prior to the rapids and they would all get out and walk around the rapids and get back in their boat at the bottom of the white water. Apparently, they had been thrown from their boat into the river along the way (imagine that). Getting thrown from the boat apparently brought up some fears for them and, in their world, the way to deal with fear was to avoid it (a typical coping strategy).

I had to explain to them that this could not continue. We were on a float trip and not a hiking expedition; all of the boats needed to stick close together for safety. I told them that most of us had families and jobs that we needed to return to before winter set in. They did manage to stay in their boat for the remainder of the float, even though their avoidance strategy may have been common to them as a family. I probably did them and the rest of the group a big favor by insisting they float down with the rest of us. Had they continued with their avoidance strategy, the white water would have become too large to face.

My good friend, Tom Davis, is the guy who is responsible for organizing the rafting trip each year. One of Tom's motivations for starting these trips was that he had a fear of water. Rather than avoiding his fear, he chose to face it. Tom's choice is dead on, and I haven't noticed him having any fear of water in a long time.

What Tom was doing is a method known as systematic desensitization, a method that is commonly used by therapists and hypnotherapists alike. In a therapeutic setting, a client would be encouraged to face their fear in baby steps. Let's say a client has agoraphobia, which is basically a fear of going out into the world. People often become confined to their own homes, because it's too uncomfortable to go out. The most extreme case that I've heard of was one I saw on a TV news program. A fellow had agoraphobia to such an extent that he locked himself in his bathroom for months and refused to come out. His wife became very creative at making foods (flatbread and pizza I would guess) that she could slip under the door. Psychologists eventually came in to work with him.

If a therapist was working with someone with agoraphobia (one of the issues when a house call may be justified), the systematic desensitization might start with the client simply imagining turning the door knob or opening the door. In following sessions the client might actually turn the door knob, or even open the door. Later sessions would have the client walking out to the mailbox to get the mail. Eventually the client would get in the car and one day drive to the grocery store. This system can take a long time to get the client back to a normal state of functioning. And this does not mean they are free of the fear, but at least they are functioning.

I watched a therapist on TV who had a group of people she was working with who shared a fear of escalators. They started off meeting as a group and talking about their issue (some guided visualization may have been involved). Later sessions included going to a department store and observing the escalator. As time went on, the group members would actually get on the escalator. Group support is a good idea in this type of situation. Seeing one person overcome his or her fear only helps to support the others in overcoming their fears as well. This type of systematic desensitization is useful, even though it can take a long time, depending on the individual involved. Those people who were part of the preceding examples were probably encouraged to continue between sessions, doing such things as opening the door on their own, or going to the department store and noticing the escalator.

In hypnosis we use systematic desensitization as well, but the process can happen much more quickly during the hypnotic trance. As you will recall in my example of the young lady with a fear of wrists, the first place I regressed her to was a happy carefree time when she was being very active. This serves several purposes: It allows the client to experience time travel in a non-threatening manner (reducing possible resistance); it gets the client in touch with their ability to experience different senses in trance; it may connect them to their point of reference (a time when they felt better about themselves); and it gives us a place to retreat for systematic desensitization. (The special place can also be used this way, but I tend to reserve it for special situations.)

After a client has been regressed to the happy, carefree time, the therapist could then regress them to an uncomfortable situation that has to do with their issue (not likely to be the ISE). When the client gets into their uncomfortable feelings, the therapist then takes them back to the happy scene. When the client experiences the happy feelings, the therapist then takes them back to the uncomfortable scene. When the client feels the discomfort, the therapist takes them back to the happy scene and gets them in touch with the good feelings. This emotional ping-pong can go back and forth for some time. Each time the uncomfortable scene is revisited, the uncomfortable feelings associated with it should become diminished. (Using a SUDs level before and after is good.) Obviously, we're not reframing the client's ISE, but we are helping the client to gain some relief.

Therapists should be aware of this type of system even if it's not their main line of therapy. This can be a way to work with a client who is resistant. It can be a way to diminish anxiety so that the client can move ahead more easily, or, if time is too short to do a full regression, this might be a viable option.

A form of desensitization also occurs when we give our clients an action plan to do between sessions (homework). Their assignments should relate to what has gone on during their session. For clients whom you've just worked with for a phobia, it's very important that they put it to the test. In the previous examples, I was able to test the clients immediately after their sessions; however, that is not always possible. Let's say someone has come to me for a fear of flying. I can't keep an airplane in my office to test them with. I could have them imagining themselves getting on the plane and check their SUDs level, which is good. Better yet, I like it if they're leaving for Chicago first thing in the morning. They'll be testing themselves right away and will be more motivated in my office to follow the process for certain success.

What if they won't be getting on a plane soon? In that case, I have them drive out to the airport and get up close and personal with the planes and situations around flying that may have been triggers in the past. This was much easier prior to 9/11. People could wander through the airport and go out onto the concourses. Now we are a bit more restricted, but people can still go to most airports and get fairly close to the action. This way they can experience that their session was successful.

This kind of testing also displays the hypnotist's confidence that his or her work is successful. If you are a therapist, then you need this kind of confidence. It is part of the waking hypnosis and you need to be confident in the process as well. If the therapist is uncertain and wishy-washy, they are not instilling confidence in the client. No matter how much knowledge you may possess as a therapist, you will not be successful until you have confidence and believe in yourself and what you are doing.

A couple of years ago I was doing a regression in front of my class as a demonstration. The young woman had a fear of elevators (more claustrophobia than anything). I took the entire class across the street to a bank building to check her SUDs level. She couldn't get on the elevator at all and was clinging to the wall. After I finished her session we went back to the bank building and she easily got on the elevator and we packed it full of students and rode to the top floor.

Another reason to test your client's success after their session is because it helps them to avoid becoming rehypnotized into their old patterns. Other people can place doubt in our client's minds and override the hypnosis we just did. Let's say we did a great session with someone who had fear of flying, we got to the ISE, and the client left our office doing great. The only problem is that this person's next flight is scheduled three months from now. If the client doesn't do something right away to prove to themselves that this really is working for them, doubt could begin to slip in. Some well meaning friend or family member might make a comment like, "I'll bet you're really dreading that flight to New York next month," or "You did hypnosis? That's never going to work." These kinds of innocent comments from others can undermine the process the client just successfully went through.

We can give suggestions in trance that any negative comment anyone else makes only strengthens the positive effects of our session (which is good). If there is to be a long period following a successful session before the client gets on an airplane, I usually suggest doing a follow-up session just prior to their departure. Another regression would probably be unnecessary, but a short interview to analyze how they are doing, and some suggestion work to reinforce the work we did, will be helpful.

While traditional systematic desensitization may seem like an easy choice, Transformational Replay is quick and gets to the core issue. If someone comes into my office and has to get on an airplane for that business trip tomorrow, I can't put them on long-term therapy.

What If You Don't Get to the ISE?

I was working with a young gentleman several years ago for a variety of issues. He was bipolar and had it under control with medication; however, he had been off his medication for a while and was experiencing some manic episodes. He had been prescribed a new fast-acting type of lithium. The doctor was to test his blood to make sure he was getting the proper dose in his system. The blood testing was a big issue for my client. He told me that any time he had blood drawn he would pass out. He wanted me to help him get over this debilitating issue.

I approached his issue in much the same manner as I have many others, including the young woman with the fear of wrists. Eventually I regressed him back to a time when he was about ten years old. His mother had a lot of emotional issues and she had been problematic throughout his life. She was getting drugs (pain killers) from some guy at a bar. My client found out what she was up to and told his grandmother and it seems the grandmother put the police onto the guy. My client saw his mother get a paring knife from the kitchen and then lock herself in the bedroom. She slit her wrists in the bedroom, but neither my client nor his siblings were able to get into the room to see what was going on or to do anything about it. His grandmother showed up on the scene and had a skeleton key that allowed her to get into the bedroom. My client saw the blood running from both of his mother's wrists, which caused him to feel weird sensations in his own wrists. His grandmother and sister were holding towels around her wrists until the fire and police department arrived and took her out on a stretcher. Blood had been spewing all around the house and it looked like a war zone.

Of course, during the hypnosis my client was abreacting and the whole thing was very emotional. Because this scene seemed so traumatic and had all of the elements of an ISE, I assumed that this must in fact be the cause of his fears. I helped him to transform this scene much in the same manner as with the young woman with the fear of wrists.

After my client had future paced himself (mental rehearsal) to the doctor's appointment for his blood test, I encouraged another future pace of my own suggestion (like I do with a lot of phobias). This time I had him imagine the doctor coming into the examining room with a big red clown nose on and big floppy shoes like clowns wear. He got a big kick out of it and left my office feeling confident.

A week later when he came back for his appointment, I asked him how his doctor's visit had gone. He said that everything went really well. He said that when the doctor came in he started laughing hysterically (due to the clown image I had planted in his subconscious), but when the doctor put the needle in his arm to draw some blood he fainted dead away. He needed to go back to the doctor within a few days to have his blood tested again. I regressed him back again to a time when he was about two and a half. He was in his pajamas and it was bedtime. He was all wound up and playing and didn't want to go to bed. His dad (who was also playing around) picked him up and put him on his bed. As soon as his dad tossed him onto the bed my client jumped off the bed and ran out of the room.

As my client was running through the house laughing he hit his head on the corner of a low mantle and knocked himself unconscious. Blood was gushing everywhere and people were yelling and screaming and scared. He was rushed to the emergency room. He became conscious just as they were injecting Novocain to the area of his wound. The Novocain was very painful and there was a lot of blood while he was being stitched up. We did the transforming piece around this ISE and all was well. When my client came back to see me, he said he was able to have blood drawn now and it was no problem whatsoever.

Even as traumatic as the scene was with his mother's attempted suicide, it was not the ISE. When we regress to a traumatic incident it is easy to believe that we have reached the ISE. If I had simply asked my client during the heat of the attempted suicide scene, "Have you ever felt these feelings and sensations prior to this time?" (or, "Are these familiar feelings and sensations that you recognize?"), I would have realized that it was not the ISE and would have regressed him further back. Oftentimes, as therapists, we don't want our clients to remain in that emotional place too long, so we jump into the transformational piece a bit prematurely. When we're helping our client, we'd really be doing more for them to stick with it until we are absolutely certain that we've gotten it all.

Doing the mental rehearsal or future pacing at the end of the session is a very good way to tell if we have achieved success. If, when taking the client into the future, the client still perceives him- or herself as having the same issue, there is a good chance that we did not get to the ISE. There have been times when I did get to the ISE and didn't get the desired results. When that happens I have found that on returning to the ISE an important piece there had been overlooked. At that point, I could transform it.

You might recall earlier that I said the ISE was never consciously remembered. For the most part that is true. There are times, however, when the ISE is consciously remembered, but not as the cause of anything. Several years ago I was sitting in on a student session. One of the students had been regressed back to a time when she was very young and was a flower girl in a wedding ceremony. Whatever she was saying suddenly triggered a memory of my own that I now experienced in a different way.

I am the middle child of three boys and was always raised as the "dumb one." All the eggs were put into the basket of my older brother who was the "smart one." I did struggle through school and eventually dropped out of high school. I never gave up, though, and went on to get all the education I could, including a lot of self-study. As I became involved in therapy, I began working at turning this thing about being the "dumb one" around. I tried a lot of different things including hypnosis, but no one had ever regressed me to the ISE. While I was observing my student's session, something she said about being the flower girl triggered the following memory.

When I was three and a half years old our family set out to California for a vacation. Our paternal grandmother and our aunt lived there and none of us kids had ever met them. We piled into Dad's '49 Kaiser and headed west. My two brothers and I came down with the measles on the way, which helped to raise the enjoyment level of the whole experience.

Cooling systems in cars back then were not that great and most of the cars crossing the desert—including ours—had a canvas bag filled with extra water for the radiator, hanging on the grill. We stopped at a gas station out in the desert. It was one of those gas stations with a sign that said something like "last chance for gas for the next 300 miles." While Dad was putting gas into the car, he gave me the canvas bag to refill with water and had me hang it back on the grill of the Kaiser. We were on the road again for quite some time when we began to notice that travelers going in the opposite direction were honking their horns and pointing. The light came on in Dad's head and he quickly pulled over to inspect the car. What he found was that when I had hung the canvas bag on the grill, I either didn't get it up high enough or the bag had slipped down while we were driving. Either way, it had dragged along the highway until the bottom had worn through and the water leaked out. From that moment on I was the "stupid kid" in the family. Dad went on and on about what a stupid thing I had done, and whenever the story about our trip to California was recounted to anyone, the event of the stupid kid and the canvas water bag was relived over and over again. From then on any dumb thing I did just reinforced the water bag incident.

During the student session, when that flash of memory came to me, one of the major epiphanies that occurred was this: The real fear on my dad's part was not that I was so stupid, but that he was. When that other car came down the road honking its horn, Dad's mind went right to the canvas bag on the front of the car. His big fear was that those faceless people in the other cars must think that he was awfully stupid to not know better than to hang the canvas bag in that manner. It was my dad's own fear of being stupid that got projected onto me at that moment. Certainly, if anyone had been stupid in this scene it was Dad. There is nothing wrong with giving a three-year-old a task like that to perform, but even if he's the world's smartest three-year-old, common sense would tell you to check up on him to make sure the job was done correctly. The main point of this story is that, although I did technically remember the ISE, until that moment in the student session I had never connected it to the start of anything.

11

The Language of Regression

The language of hypnotherapy is different from our everyday conscious conversational language. In hypnosis we are addressing the subconscious mind. That's not to say that the conscious mind is never present. The conscious mind uses critical, analytical, intellectual, judgmental kinds of verbiage. The conscious mind may say things like, *I don't remember,* or *I don't know,* or *this can't be right.* The subconscious is the intuitive, creative, feeling aspect of the mind and this is the part that we wish to engage for Transformational Replay. The subconscious is in the moment, feeling and experiencing what is happening. The conscious mind gives a report on what it *thinks* happened or can remember. If a client uses conscious mind language like, *I can't remember* or *I think* or *don't think,* then we need to encourage the client to be in the subconscious with suggestions, "Don't think; be there now."

Language for Regression Therapists to Avoid

Try

The word "try" implies failure. How many people have *tried* to lose weight or *tried* to stop smoking? Have you ever said, *I'll try*, if you don't really want to make it to that party or other event? If I'm regressing a client to an uncomfortable experience and I say, *Try and go back in time*, I could be met with resistance. *Try* is not *do*.

Why

This word tends to engage the conscious analytical mind and we do not want that. All questions can be asked with "what" or "how," instead of "why." Instead of, *Why do you feel that way?* one can ask, *How does that make you feel?* Instead of asking, *Why is this happening?* a therapist could query, *What's the cause of this?* or, *Talk about the cause*, or, *Explain the cause*. Even from these few examples you can begin to notice how the "why" questions only cause us to analyze and engage the conscious mind.

See

A lot of therapists use the word "see" over and over: *What do you see now? Tell me what you see. Can you see anyone?* When a therapist uses the word "see" all of the time, it's a good indicator that the therapist is visually oriented and just assumes that works for the rest of the world. Most people would probably do all right with a suggestion to *see*, but a lot of people are not visually oriented. Some people will become totally frustrated by a therapist who continually asks what they are seeing. Lots of people are auditory or kinesthetic and may not respond well to *see* commands. We can use methods to determine if someone is auditory, visual or kinesthetic or we can adjust our language to work well with whatever modality a person may prefer. Words like "notice" or "experience" are not specific to any particular sensory modality.

Remember

In regression, never ask the client to "remember." Remembering is a conscious mind activity and we do not want to engage the conscious mind. Instead of saying, *Remember when this happened to you before?* one could say, *Go back to an earlier time when you feel these similar feelings and sensations.*

Think

Like remembering, thinking is a conscious mind activity. Use, *How is it for you growing up as a poor farm boy?* instead of, *Think about how hard life must have been when you were young.*

Painted Words

Avoid using painted words. Painted words are the words that describe the issue we are trying to get away from. *Headache, pain, fear, anxiety, grief,* are a few examples of painted words. If someone has come to get rid of a headache and the therapist continually uses the word "headache," it only reinforces exactly what we don't want. A therapist could facilitate a really effective session for their client and undermine the whole session by using painted words. It is especially important to avoid painted words at the end of a session. What if the therapist just completed a successful session around headaches and as soon as the client emerges from trance the therapist says, *So how is that headache now,* or, *Is the headache gone?* In order for the client to answer that question they have to look inside for symptoms of a headache and, lo and behold, there it is! Avoid any language (script) that continually uses painted words. Consider using something like, *These new feelings and sensations are so much better than something else.*

Pharsing

Pharsing is a phenomenon that occurs when we use words of a *not* derivative such as *can't, don't, won't, shouldn't, couldn't, wouldn't,* and the like. When we begin a statement with a word that is a *not* derivative, the mind tends only to hear what follows it. If I say, *Don't think of the Eiffel Tower,* what do you think about? If one of my boys is running out the back door and I say, *Don't slam the screen door,* his mind only hears, *Slam the screen door!* At times, we can use pharsing in our favor, such as, *You probably don't notice how relaxed you're feeling,* or, *You probably wouldn't enjoy going out with me.* However, for the most part, don't use don't.

Past Tense

The therapist's language should not be in past tense: *What was it like when you were abandoned? How old were you back then?* If your client is in the subconscious, then they are in the now, which is different than where the therapist is in the present moment. The therapist talking in past tense may draw the client back into the conscious mind.

I want you to …

I want you to and its cousins, *I would like you to,* or *I need you to* is unnecessary language. When a therapist says, *I want you to,* it's drawing the focus away from the client and toward the therapist. The more defiant client may internally respond with, *What do I care about what you want?* There is also the ego of the therapist involved in *I want you to.* Many, many scripts open with the words, *I want you to,* and that doesn't make it all right. As hypnotists, the main tool we have to work with is our voice. How we use that instrument should be carefully considered. A lot of purpose and thought needs to be placed into the verbiage that passes from our lips. Simply eliminating the words, *I want you to,* and its variations, helps to make every statement work better. Notice if I say, *I want you to go back to a time when blah, blah happened.* Then hear the same statement without the personal inflection: *Go back to a time that blah, blah happened.* Notice the difference? Eliminate *I want you to* from your hypnotic language.

Monotone

It was common in years gone by for the hypnotist to speak in a monotone and some still do. Monotone can actually be effective when the conscious mind is present and the hypnotist is trying to lull the mind into hypnosis. However, when we are working with the subconscious mind, the therapist needs to put more life into their language. *How* we say something can be as important as *what* we say (intention). If I were to use a very Eeore-the-donkey-like voice and say, *Experience your mother standing right in front or you,* it will not evoke the same response as it will if I put some real intensity and intention into my voice. ***Experience your mother standing in front of you right now! What do you need to say to Mother?***

Permissive Language

Some therapists are way too permissive with their language. Being permissive is fine when we're dealing with the conscious mind, but we are addressing the subconscious mind with Transformational Replay. By saying something like, *You can go back in time when you're ready,* or, *You can go back whenever you feel like it,* the therapist is using statements that are a lot like using the word "try." The therapist may be regressing his or her client back to an emotional event. The mind is aware that this could be uncomfortable and, by using permissive language, the therapist has just given the client a way to avoid moving ahead. Permissive language will not cut it with regression. Being directive will get our clients to their healing much more quickly. I have watched too many sessions drift off into the ozone because permissive language did not keep the client on track. In my opinion, it is not all right for hypnotists to just say, *That's where the subconscious needed to go for now.* We, as therapists, need to keep our client on track and achieve the goal that we are after, rather than subjecting our clients to endless sessions of drifting around in fairyland.

Language That Therapists Should Use

Present Tense

The therapist's language should always be in the present tense. Your client is in the subconscious mind and in the moment. Keep your client in the moment. Use wording like, *What's happening now? What are you feeling? Are you alone or with someone? How does that make you feel? How old are you now?*

Simple Language

Use simple language. Avoid big flowery words and esoteric terms. Complicated language will only serve to engage the client's conscious mind and draw them away from their trance experience. Language of about an eighth grade level is fine.

Intensity or Animation

The therapist's voice and language help to keep the session moving in the direction we need to go. Avoid using the monotone. Be expressive as is necessary. The subconscious works well with drama and enthusiasm. I recommend that my students read children's books out loud to each other. Books like *The Three Little Pigs* have lots of good energy in the content and, because of the simple language, we can read it without getting hung up on the words. This helps us to build confidence to speak similarly in a session. Acting lessons and storytelling classes would be useful as well. Practice reading out loud or into a tape recorder. Listen to your voice. Do you feel convinced by your own words?

Directive Language

When doing Transformational Replay, we need to keep our clients on track. Directive language helps to keep the client moving along in the proper direction. I've witnessed too many regressions, done in a permissive style, that wander all over until the goal of the session is lost. Often the therapist will say that the subconscious mind just needed to go there (wherever it is they have allowed the client to wander) and we will continue working towards the goal next week. With directive language the therapist can keep the session more goal oriented. Directive language keeps the session and the client on task. Use words like, *Go back, back to an earlier time when you feel these same feelings and sensations!* or, *Go back to the very first time you feel these same feelings and sensations!*

Phrases to Repeat

The following statements are what I refer to as the short course to regression therapy. Using these simple phrases over and over will get you a long way:

- "That's right ..."
- "What's happening now?"
- "What happens next?"
- "How does that make you feel?"
- "Where do you notice these feelings and sensations in your body?"
- "That's right ..."

"That's right ..." This can be very subtle, but very important, and that's why I've repeated it. When a client is moving in the proper direction, a subtle *That's right* can encourage them to continue. If I notice my client taking a breath or sighing as they slip deeper into trance, a gentle *That's right* will help to encourage them. Also, it helps to train them to be a good client. If I notice some emotion starting, again a subtle *That's right* will let them know they're okay and doing well. Occasionally, *Thaaaaat's riiiight* can work also.

At times, *That's right* may not be so subtle to bring the client more into the moment. Use, **That's right, the SOB is hurting you!** or, **That's right, you're very upset; you feel angry!** By emphasizing the words the client has just given you, you may also be reassuring and encouraging the client into his or her true emotions.

"What's happening now?" This is a simple directive statement that lets the therapist know where their client is. A variation is, *Give a report.*

"What happens next?"   This helps to move the client ahead while staying in the same time period. Sometimes, a sense of urgency in the therapist's voice can help the client move ahead and remain in their current feelings.

"How does that make you feel?"   This helps to get the client in touch with their feelings and also helps the therapist to create the affect bridge.

"Where do you notice these feelings and sensations in your body?" This helps us to create the affect bridge as well. Often the therapist will notice that the areas where the client notices emotional sensations in their body are also the areas that will shift to new positive sensations once we have transformed the ISE. Be sure to make notes about these feelings and sensations as they occur and underline them. As the therapist you may think you will remember everything as the session progresses, but I wouldn't rely on that. If the session needs to end prior to reaching the ISE, it will be much easier to get right back to where you were in following sessions. Later, when you are reviewing your notes, the notes will make more sense with the added detail.

12

Go Back to the Very First Time

W hen doing Transformational Replay the statement, is an inevitable one. It might sound something like, *Go back, back to the very first time you feel these feelings and sensations!* This statement can lead to some very interesting discoveries, as in the following.

I was working with a young woman who was here from another country doing studies. She was an avid student of Buddhism and a dedicated meditator. She had been using her studies to help deal with her past. She progressed very well with her hypnosis sessions. After I said, *Go back to the very first time you feel these feelings and sensations,* this is what followed:

Client: I'm watching my mother in her bedroom. She's upset and crying. (*My client has not yet been conceived.*) Her father has confined her to her room. It's Saturday night and mother wants to go out. She's very pretty and her father doesn't trust her and he's afraid she will get into trouble.

Me: What happens next?

Client: Mother waits until it's late and climbs out of her bedroom window. She goes to a club and goes dancing.

Me: Then what happens?

Client: She dances until late at night. She meets a man that she's having a lot of fun with.

Me: What happens next?

Client: They're climbing in her bedroom window. She doesn't want to do anything, but he is very insistent. Mother is very scared. She doesn't want to get caught. I am the result of this encounter.

Me: What happens next?

Client: Days go by ... Mother is noticing things about her body. She's very worried. She realizes she must be pregnant.

Me: Then what happens?

Client: More time goes by ... She's terrified of what will happen. Finally, she tells her mother. Her mother is very upset and rushes her to the doctor. Too much time has gone by ... it's too late for an abortion. Together they decide to keep the pregnancy a secret as long as possible.

Me: What happens next?

Client: They manage to keep it a secret for quite some time, but eventually her father gets wise and throws a fit. She's crying and terrified. (*Client is emoting.*) Her father banishes her from the house.

Me: What's happening now?

Client: It's dark and cold. (*emoting*) Mom is sitting out on a park bench crying and scared. There's nowhere to go, no one to turn to.

Me: Then what happens?

Client: It's three or four A.M. Her mother comes out to the park bench. She sneaks my mother inside and hides her in the house. At least she's inside for now.

Me: Then what happens?

Client: The next day her mother convinces her father to let her stay in the back of the house. Mother has to stay out of his sight or he'll throw her back out. He's mean and angry and can get violent. Her mom is very afraid of him also. He can do bad things.

Me: What happens next?

Client: Time goes by and it's awful being secluded, but at least Mother is inside and relatively safe.

Me: Then what happens?

Client: We're in the hospital. Mom's scared. People are all around. There's lots of confusion. I'm scared! I come out into the bright lights. It's cold. I get swept up and carried away. I'm all wrapped up. Someone is carrying me away. I'm scared! (*The client is writhing in agony and emoting.*)

Me: What's happening now?

Client: Where's my mommy? I want my mommy! Someone's taking me away! Mommy was crying out to me! Where's my mommy?

Me: What's happening now?

Client: I'm in a room with a lot of other babies. There's the sound of crying, sometimes it's me and sometimes other babies. Where's my mother?

Me: What happens next?

Client: It's horrible. I'm in this room full of other babies for several days and no mommy.

Me: Then what happens?

Client: Someone takes me away to another room. There's my mother! She takes me and holds me. I grab her finger and I hold on for dear life. She looks at me and says, "I'll never let anything happen to you again." I feel much better. I won't let go of her finger.

Of course we did a transformational piece around this whole regression and I will talk about that further in the text. First I will fill in some vital information.

The promise that my client's mother made to her to never let anything happen to her was short lived. She was given away to another family to raise. My client was a black child. Her mother was white. The part of Europe where they lived at the time had almost no black people. The young man that my client's mother encountered at the night club was an American GI who was stationed there temporarily. Her family was Catholic and the nuns in the hospital assumed that, because this was a black child to a white unwed mother, it must have been going up for adoption. Her parents may have allowed them to believe that as well. That is why the baby was kept in the nursery for three days before she got to see her mother. Her mother had wanted her and had tried to convince the staff of that, but it took three days before they finally believed her and brought the child in.

Mother and child came home for only a short time until the parents arranged for another family to raise the child. My client was raised in a situation where she was treated poorly. Her adoptive brothers and sisters were treated much differently than she was. She had to struggle to make it and was shown very little attention or affection. Her birth mother had moved away from home and went on to make a living as stripper and a call girl.

How can we possibly know all of this? It just so happens that, at the same time that I'm doing hypnotherapy with my client, her mother is in Europe doing hypnotherapy as well, and trying to straighten out her awful past. My client's mother had also made contact with her, wanting to create a new relationship and heal their past.

When my client described what had gone on in her hypnosis session, her mother verified everything almost word for word. She told my client that when the nuns brought her into her hospital room, "You grabbed onto my finger and held on for dear life," and I said, "I'll never let anything ever happen to you." She also said, "What are we going to do now?"

How can this be? How could an unborn child, especially a child that hasn't been conceived yet, have awareness of what was happening in the world? Could it be that some family members or someone had related these events at some point? Certainly the adoptive parents were not privy to this kind of information. My client had some contact with her mother as a child, but it was quite brief and she was very young. Could she have consciously or subconsciously remembered something that had been related to her that far back? Is it possible that she was actually able to tap into some memory or psychic ability that allowed her access to this information? I don't know the answers to any of these questions. I do know, though, that during the many years I have worked with hypnosis, things have occurred that I can't explain. All I know is that my client experienced healing during this session and that is the part that is important to me. I also know that my client's mother did verify what occurred during our session.

Perhaps the happy ending to this whole piece is that my client's mother did quite well over the years in her chosen profession. She bought a nice home and settled down to retire and straighten her life out. My client moved back to Europe to live with her and work their lives out together. Let's hope for the best for them. This is where the statement, *Go back to the very first time you have these feelings and sensations,* can lead!

A young woman came into my office trying to resolve her issues of abandonment and unexplained anger. Her session follows:

Me: Go back, back in time to the very first time you feel these feelings and sensations.

Client: I'm floating, it's dark. I'm warm; I feel pressure on my shoulders and on the outside of my arms. I don't feel anything touching me.

Me: What else?

Client: Sad. I feel sad, heavy. My chest is heavy, it's hard to breathe. I feel hopeless, trapped, confined.

Me: How old are you? (*I suspect she may be in the womb.*)

Client: I don't know how old, I can't talk or see. I can't feel anything. It's warm.

Me: Anything else?

Client: I'm sad, heavy heart. I feel anger. I feel a weight. I'm in someone. I'm not born yet. My mother is angry. She's been very angry about something for a long time. It makes me angry. It makes me sad. I don't know what she's angry about, she's angry a lot. I feel sad, I feel angry. I'm reflecting her pain.

Me: Now what?

Client: Trapped!

Me: What happens next?

Client: Cold now. Hands, arms are cold, circulation is poor. Outside, it's cold. I can breathe better now. I had to get out, had to change. Don't be stuck. Do something, move.

Me: What next?

Client: Now rocking. Being rocked. Someone is rocking me. No touch. No human warmth. Back and forth motion like I'm being rocked. Hands are tiny and cold.

Me: What next?

Client: Rocking again. I can't tell who's got me. Not happy. No joy. Don't know where mother is. Lots of tears. I don't want to be alone. Don't want to be with anyone. No one is here. It's okay. Don't like it. I'll go away.

This is one of the rare times when the client went straight to the ISE. I've had it happen from time to time, but don't count on it. This was the first time I had worked with this person. It's really time efficient when this happens, but it's rare. Of course, we did a transformational piece and again I will discuss that further in the text.

What came out of this session was that my client had picked up her unexplained anger in utero. Her mother was very angry while she was carrying my client and the unborn child was picking up on the anger. I believe the mother also had post-partum depression, which only exacerbated the anger and abandonment feelings for my client. The person who was rocking her was either someone in the nursery or her mother being very detached due to the post-partum depression.

When my client came in to see me she reported that she had a good childhood and there had been no trauma or abuse. She couldn't understand why she was having these feelings. You might think that this womb experience is unusual or made up. However, I find this not to be so unusual at all. Many times when I have regressed a client back to an ISE, it ends up being a birth or in utero experience. It was commonly believed that the newborn or unborn child has no awareness, and was treated accordingly. In my practice, it has been proven to me over and over that we do have consciousness. Perhaps that consciousness is not the same as we experience later in life; however, I am convinced that we do have consciousness.

Many times when I have regressed someone back to the origin of anxiety or abandonment issues, we have accessed a birth or in utero experience. Even the best situations can go awry. Let's say a young couple is very much in love. They have planned their pregnancy and have been looking forward to the birth of their child. Even in an ideal situation such as this, complications can occur. The unborn child could be wrapped in the cord or be a breech delivery. There are any number of possibilities. What if the child is premature, or some other complication causes the baby to go into surgery, or be kept in an incubator, or in a nursery, isolated from its mother? Even with the best parents and the best intentions problems can occur. What about those babies who are born into situations that are less than ideal? What if the child is completely unwanted or the product of extremely dysfunctional or low functioning individuals? What about those individuals who were never wanted at all and were given up for adoption? It shouldn't be too difficult to see how these scenarios could lead to issues later in life.

My wife, Lynsi, does a lot of work in the area of HypnoFertility and HypnoBirthing. These processes provide a much gentler birthing experience. I've witnessed these newly born tiny babies reaching out to Lynsi the first time they hear her voice. I am convinced that those babies have become aware of her gentle verbiage while in utero and that they recognize her. I encourage my clients to talk to their unborn children. It really does seem to have a positive effect.

Just prior to our birth we have more neurons in the brain that at any other time in our life. The reason for that is uncertain. There's a good possibility that having all of those extra neurons helps to build in redundancy. There are certain functions that are so important to our survival that the body overcompensates just to make sure that these functions do occur. Could it be possible that this excess of neurons is also helping us to better sense our surroundings? Perhaps we have more awareness in utero than we think.

My experience has shown me that the unborn baby is picking up on the emotions of its parents, and, obviously, the mother's emotions would be very apparent to the baby. This was the case in the previous example. My client's unexplained anger was really anger that she had picked up from her mother. It would be difficult for a mother to avoid every possible emotional situation; however, we can make the best of any situation. If some negative situation occurs, we can relax and talk with the unborn child and explain and give comfort. It's good to explain that this is a temporary thing. Tell the baby how much you are looking forward to greeting it and relating to it in a whole new way. Let the baby know that there are other people (family and friends) waiting to play a role in its life.

What if I'm completely wrong? What if the unborn and newborn child has no consciousness of any sort? If that is the case, would it be so horrible to treat that unborn or newly born baby with love and caring regardless of what we might believe?

13

The Ethics of Regression

The use of hypnosis to lead a client into an awareness of unpleasant experiences *must* be based on the belief that reliving a particular experience will be worthwhile and beneficial to the client. Academic psychology has taught students that reliving unpleasant experiences makes them less harmful—*not so!* The reality is that if a particular set of experiences teaches a particular response, then going through the same experiences again only serves to reinforce what was learned from those particular experiences. If what was learned created limitations in the person, reliving the event over again in the same way serves to reinforce the generalizations. Fortunately, with the Transformational Replay technique, clients have the opportunity to recreate those emotions, in order to have a new and empowering outcome. For clients who have been brutalized or abused, it would likely be particularly harmful for them to experience that particular trauma without transforming it.

The caveat to this is that oftentimes when the client and therapist reach the ISE, there is the "AHA! Experience." That is, the light comes on for the client, they see the cause of their symptoms, and the symptoms disappear in that moment. This is what hypnotists have often relied on in the past. Academic psychology would be revisiting the SSEs and not the ISE, so it is unlikely that a core issue would ever get resolved. Without reframing these incidents, the client is likely to become more traumatized, feel that they or their therapy is failing, and are likely to give up. Oftentimes, when I have worked with clients who have had previous therapy, they will say, *Yeah, I've already dealt with that*, or, *I've been there and it didn't help and I don't want to go back.* This may prevent me from being able to help them. Other times when I do regress one of these clients, they are amazed at what they hadn't accomplished in those other sessions, and that what they thought was the cause of their issue was really something else that they were unaware of.

I believe there are times when therapists get to an ISE, actually transform it, and aren't even aware of what they have achieved. This is more likely to occur in Gestalt work and other emotionally based processes. It's not very likely that traditional types of talk therapy would be able to stumble into an ISE, because talk therapy is much more cognitive.

The rule of thumb is: Don't regress your client to a trauma, unless you are going to reframe the scenario in a better way. Even if you have not reached the ISE and need to end wherever you are, the outcome should be transformed.

What About False Memory?

False memory is not a real thing. *Planted memory* might be a better way to describe it. Not so many years back, you may have heard about false memory syndrome. People were sued and families were broken up over situations that never occurred. Most of these problems were caused by therapists who had their own agenda. Many of these therapists may have themselves suffered from some form of abuse. If their client then demonstrated any symptoms that could have had a similar origin, the therapist projected that similar abuse right into the client's session. If I say to my client, *See the Eiffel Tower,* the mind has no problem going there. The client may have never been to the Eiffel Tower; however, we've all seen pictures of the tower or can at least imagine in our minds what it must be like. Okay, no problem so far. However, what if I have my own agenda and now I say, *See your father raping you!* Again the mind has no problem going there. Does that mean it happened? Does that mean it's any more real than the Eiffel Tower? Some therapists encouraged their clients to believe that this was real and that they had just uncovered a hidden memory.

Some therapists encouraged their clients to confront their perpetrator and take legal action. This is not good. It is very important that therapists stay impartial, no matter what kind of therapy we are doing. In my opinion, any memory that comes from regression (other than for forensic purposes) should be thought of as metaphorical, even though it may be very real. It could be difficult, or even impossible, to prove the evidence that was uncovered in trance. If we pursue the trance experience and confront a perpetrator, it could all get very messy, and that could serve to make the client's life even worse. Our client's healing and well-being should be our primary goal, rather than punishing the perpetrators.

Years ago it was fashionable to confront our abusers, but too often these confrontations ruined families. I know of cases where perpetrators have attempted to atone for their wrongdoings, but that is rare. Most perpetrators will go into denial about what occurred, or they will lie, or in some other way avoid the truth. After all, what kind of person could do such a thing? Only someone who was mentally ill could have done such a thing, and who would want to admit to being crazy? So now their back is against the wall. And the only easy way out is denial.

My older brother confronted my father a number of times about the abuse that occurred in his childhood. This confrontation only served to drive a wedge between the two of them. Dad just went further and further into denial. They wouldn't speak to each other for years on end and there was a lot of anger and animosity between them. I got to be the middleman.

At one point my father was coming into town and my brother told me that he was going to confront him once and for all, this time in front of me. This seemed to him like a good plan. I explained to my brother that whenever he had confronted Dad in the past, it was just the two of them, which left Dad with an out. Dad could always go into denial, because no one else was present to verify what the truth was. With me present, Dad would no longer have an out. That would put Dad under a great deal of pressure because his usual avoidance tactics would now be useless. I explained to my brother that Dad was very old and probably only had a few years left. Dad was also not very stable and, if backed against the wall, might take extraordinary measures to deal with the situation. I asked my brother if he would feel better if Dad took his life after being confronted about the past? I told my brother that he was more emotionally stable than Dad, and it would be more productive to help him improve his quality of life rather than to take away the little time that Dad had left on earth.

Often the victims of abuse feel that if they can just get back at the abuser (cause them to feel the same pain that they have felt), somehow this will cause them to feel better. Regardless of whether that would be beneficial or not, the truth is that the other person is not likely to feel the way we would want them to, nor are they likely to make the connection between what they are feeling and what happened to the victim. Even if the abuser were to hurt in the way that the victim hopes, and even if they connected that to their actions, it's still unlikely that the victim would feel the satisfaction he or she had hoped for. In the end, I believe it's better to heal ourselves through our own inner work.

There are times, of course, when abuse or other things have occurred, and it can and should be proven and acted on through legal means. Things like child abuse need to be nipped in the bud whenever possible. Far too many bad things have happened to people. There is no need for therapists to invent more.

14

The Process—In a Nutshell

Step One

Intake: to get the client's personal information and history and to create the session intention.

Along with your normal intake, the following are some other things to discuss:

- Find out what medications the client might be on. Some medications can have a negative effect on the hypnosis session. Some medications may have side effects that are causing or worsening the client's issue(s). If you feel that a medication may be interfering with the hypnosis, you may resolve this issue by adjusting the time of the appointment to coincide with a time when the side effects of the medications are less apparent.

- Were there any traumas to the client growing up (accidents, surgeries, someone close to them dying, or the like)? These may be SSEs related to the client's issue.

- Was there any abuse (physical, emotional, sexual)?

- What does the client know about their birth? Was it late, early, breech, C-section, or were there other complications? Were they kept in an incubator or nursery? These things can be the beginning of anxiety or abandonment issues.

- What has the client come in for (perhaps it's a phobia)?

- When was the first time the client was aware of the presenting issue? Most likely your client will recall an SSE or something that a family member has brought to their attention.

- Has there ever been a time when this wasn't an issue (for point of reference)? If we functioned in the world without this issue in the past, we can do it again.

- When was the most recent time this was an issue? This relates to Step Four of the process. This helps us to create the affect bridge.

Listen carefully to what your client has to say. Have them describe what they feel when their issue is occurring. When your client describes the sensations that they notice, like a knot in the stomach, or shortness of breath, or their throat closes up, these are sensations that help you to create the affect bridge. You will be able to use this information later in trance.

Take good notes. You may think you can remember things that your client is saying, but in the middle of a session, when things are moving fast, you'll be glad to have your notes to fall back on. Underline emotions and body sensations that are going to help you to create the affect bridge. In addition, underline things that the client says you can feed back to them as direct suggestions at the end of their session.

If this is the first time you have seen this client, it will be necessary to thoroughly explain the hypnotic process and the difference between the conscious and subconscious mind. The conscious mind is the analytical, critical, judgmental, intellectual mind. The subconscious is the intuitive, feeling, creative mind.

If you will be doing an induction that includes body manipulation, like the *Elman arm drop*, let your client know about this so that they will not be startled if you lift their arm during trance.

I often use the thump and bump method of tapping the client on the forehead to access the subconscious mind (a la Jerry Kein). You need to let your client know about this prior to trance, so as not to startle them out of trance (more on this method later). Also, let your client know that you may, at some point, be asking them to make up a story. Explain that when we ask them to make up a story, it's not to create fiction; the purpose is to engage the subconscious mind. The conscious mind does not make up stories. The conscious mind will give us reports or opinions and judgments. Only the subconscious can make up the story. This helps us to get back into the subconscious mind and move ahead.

Make certain to let the client know that the feelings they are experiencing may be feelings that are triggered by the situation (fear of flying, for example), and that the actual cause of these feelings may have nothing to do with flying at all (more likely it's a fear of losing control, or claustrophobia, or the like). But if you take the client back to the first time they flew on a plane and then take them back further, the conscious mind might interfere because it seems irrational since they never flew in a plane prior to this time. If they are aware in the beginning that it is the origin of the emotions that we are looking for and not the situation that is currently connected with these feelings, then the client will be more likely to keep moving smoothly through the process.

It's also important that the therapist explains that he or she will be asking questions in trance and that the client will be giving answers. Unless the client is aware that they will be talking, they may not expect to answer questions, which can startle them and cause them to come out of trance.

Step Two

Do an induction to the client's safe place. I like to use the stairs because it gives some nice opportunities to reaffirm the session intention. Whatever induction method the therapist chooses should be strong and effective. We need to achieve somnambulism. Without proper induction, some therapists only get their client into light hypnosis and may experience resistance or achieve only a pseudo regression. Often the client who gets into an emotional state will go into somnambulism because of the emotions; however, their therapist is often unaware that this has occurred. As the therapist, don't count on emotions pulling the client into somnambulism, because if you don't get the emotions there's a good chance that you won't get them into somnambulism after the process begins.

When the therapist has taken the client to their safe place, have them fully describe what they are experiencing. Have them notice their various senses and anchor the good feelings with their breath. (*Take in a deep breath and breathe in these good feelings and sensations.*) This helps to establish the safe place and also shows them that they can interact while in hypnosis in an easy non-threatening way.

Some therapists may think I take too much time getting into the work. I find that I very rarely fail to get my client to the ISE in that first session. If I used other methods (which I have done) I might fail to achieve our goal and then it doesn't really matter how much time I saved.

Step Three

This step is done to show the client that they can travel back in time in a non-threatening way. If the therapist jumps right into some emotional event in the past, the client's defenses are likely to come up. Once we have successfully taken them back in time to an event, they will be unable to say they can't do that. This can help to speed up the process considerably. The therapist needs to be like the detective, Jack Webb, by always sticking to the facts with questioning. I've watched students get off on tangents, asking things like, "Are those pants corduroy?" or, "It's the fifties; are you in a Chevy, or maybe it's a '56 Ford?" This type of questioning is totally unnecessary and will get the regression off track, causing the client to engage their conscious mind and/or lighten the trance state.

Take the client back to a happy, carefree time, an active time. (This could be the client's point of reference depending on what you are working on.) This needs to be a pleasant experience that we can return to if necessary. The reason I like to choose an active time is because it helps to integrate more of the senses, and I like to encourage more exercise wherever possible.

After the safe place, use this wording:

> In a moment I'm going to ask you to go back in time and you will go back in time, you will go back to a happy, carefree time, a time when you are being very active, perhaps you're involved in some sporting event as a youngster, or some childhood game, or some other activity which causes you to use your body in a vigorous manner. It's a happy time, a carefree time. So, now take a deep breath and feel yourself drifting back to that happy, carefree, active time.

Ask the client to respond. *Tell me what you see or feel.* Usually the client will start right in. However, if they hesitate, jump in with, *First impressions! Indoors or out?* Allow a brief pause for the client to respond. Repeat the statement if necessary. *Alone or with someone?* Say these phrases without hesitation and you will engage the subconscious mind.

The client will usually begin with something like, *It's a late summer evening. A bunch of us neighborhood kids are running through the yards. Kids are laughing and yelling.*

Therapist: How old are you?

Client: I'm eight years old.

Therapist: What are you wearing?

Client: I'm wearing cut off jean shorts and a tank top and my New York Yankees baseball cap. (*This helps to show the client that they can bring things out in trance that would not be possible through conscious memory.*)

Therapist: What's happening?

Client: We're playing hide and seek.

Therapist: How does that make you feel?

Client: It's exciting! We're running and screaming through the neighborhood. The night air is exhilarating.

Therapist: Notice your young eight-year-old muscles, so strong, so limber, so full of energy. It feels like you can go on and on forever. Notice other sensations like the excitement in the air, the energy, so happy, so carefree. With each breath, you breathe in these good, happy, carefree sensations, deep into every cell of your body. More and more, these are the good feelings and sensations you notice, more and more. More and more, it feels good to use your body in a physical manner. More and more, it feels good to experience these happy carefree sensations.

Now we have trained our client to travel in time and we have encouraged good feelings and physical activity. Also we have created a place to come back to that can be used for hypnotic systematic desensitization, if we should need it.

Step Four

This step starts to move the client back in time toward their ISE, and it's relatively easy since it was just the other day.

Here the therapist takes the client to a recent time, perhaps the most recent time, that the client had an experience with their issue. (Let's use a phobia, like fear of flying, for instance.) This is not going to be an ISE because it just happened recently. Most likely they will be connecting with an SIE (symptom intensifying event).

It is important to make good use of the Step Four portion of the regression. It can quickly get the client in touch with the emotions that are associated with the ISE. This will help us to create the affect bridge that is our ticket to the ISE.

Encourage the client to be in the moment, to be in the feelings. It is important that the therapist use directive language; the sense of urgency that the therapist uses throughout the regression is more important than the exact wording. If the client uses language like,

What I remember is, or, *What I think happened is …* jump right in with, *Not "remember," be there now, what is happening now, what are you feeling now?* If the client starts to speak in the past tense, get them in the moment. Say something like, *Not back then; what's happening now? Be in the moment! What are you feeling now? Where do you feel these sensations in your body now?* This helps to keep the client in their subconscious mind where they need to be.

A Step Four portion of the regression goes something like this (after completion of Step Three):

Therapist: Now take a deep breath and feel yourself drifting back in time, back to a recent time, perhaps the most recent time, that you noticed difficulties around flying in airplanes.

This method of using the breath to create transitions has served me well; however, I have done thousands of these regressions and have become very comfortable with moving clients along in this manner. People may be more comfortable using a one-two-three count, such as, "In a moment I will count from one to three. When I reach the count of three you will be at a recent time, perhaps the most recent time, that this fear of flying was apparent. One … two … three … Be there now. It's a recent time, perhaps the most recent time, that you have this fear of flying!" If you should use the breath as I do, be certain not to tell the client to relax after you tell him or her to take a deep breath. As hypnotists, we often become used to saying, "Take a deep breath and relax." However, in this case, we do not want our clients to relax. We want to keep them in their current emotions. Whichever method you choose, it's important to create consistency. We are creating a transition each time, but we are also creating an expectancy within the client that we are moving into something new. The smoother and more consistent and confident the therapist is, the more the client is being trained to be a good client.

Client: It's last Wednesday, I'm driving to the airport.

Therapist: What are you noticing?

Client: (*Squirming in the chair and the client's breathing has become erratic*)
My palms are sweaty, my breathing is heavy and restricted, I've got this
huge knot in my stomach, and I feel panicky just thinking about the
plane flight.

At this point the therapist could continue moving the client further into this scene. This might be necessary, especially if the client
hasn't fully gotten into the emotions around this event. Perhaps it
might take going down the concourse or actually boarding the plane,
or maybe the engines need to start up, or perhaps the actual takeoff
needs to occur to trigger the emotions that will create the affect
bridge. In this particular case, the client is already writhing in their
seat and their breathing shows signs of panic. The knot in the stomach was described to the therapist during the intake and that is significant. Even though we have not ventured far into Step Four, the
therapist has all of the elements to create the affect bridge. These
feelings from Step Four will take us all the way to the ISE.

The mission of Step Four is to lay the groundwork that will get
us back to the ISE. There is no need to do any transformational
(reframing) pieces until we've finished with the ISE or have to end
the session prior to reaching the ISE. I like to avoid sending a client
out the door after being in the middle of some emotional event; so
even if the session isn't complete it's good to salvage as much as possible. This may be all it takes to resolve the issue.

Step Five

*The fifth step will most likely get them in touch with another SIE, the
SPE, or an SSE.*

Occasionally a client might go straight to an ISE (as in the earlier
example), but it's not likely. It is much more likely that Step Five will
be repeated a number of times before the client reaches the ISE.

Take the client back in time to an earlier time when this incident
occurred (fear of flying) or they feel these similar feelings and sensations. It's best if the client is still feeling the sensations like the

erratic breathing, sweaty palms and the knot in the stomach, while the therapist is transitioning them to Step Five. If, during the Step Four portion, the client moved to a segment of the scene where the emotions dissipated, then move them back into the emotive portion. It's easier to move the client back with the affect bridge while the client is still feeling the emotions.

Therapist: Take a deep breath (*or count one, two, three*) and move back in time, back to an earlier time, when you experience these same feelings and sensations. Be there now. What's happening now? (*If there is hesitation then quickly say, "First impressions, indoors or out? Alone or with someone?"*)

Client: I'm on that flight to Seattle; it's December of '98; I had just gotten married that week and I am upset that the company is sending me away from home so soon. It's almost Christmas, I need to do my shopping, and I hate being gone.

Therapist: What happens next?

Client: I've been worrying about my new bride and the plane is bouncing around. I've been in turbulence before, but this is worse, people are screaming, things are moving around in the cabin.

Therapist: What are you feeling?

Client: I'm scared to death! We're going to crash! I'm going to die! My heart is racing, I can't breathe, my stomach is all knotted up. (*The client is writhing in the chair, gripping and clutching at the furniture.*) I'll never see my wife again!

Therapist: Have you ever felt these feelings and sensations prior to this moment? (*If there is any hesitation, use, "Do you recognize these feelings and sensations," or, "Are these new feelings and sensations that you've never had before?"*)

Client: Yes.

Therapist: Go back, back, back in time, to an earlier time that you feel these same or similar sensations, the shortness of breath, the knot in your stomach, back, back in time. What's happening now?

Client: Oh no! It's my girl friend, Judy. She's riding down Main Street with my best friend Steve! She's sitting next to him and his arm is around her! We were getting along just fine. This can't be!

Therapist: What are you feeling?

Client: There's that knot in my stomach, I can hardly breathe, it must be some mistake. I rush over to Judy's house later that day. I'm scared to death, but I hope I was wrong about what I saw. She tells me she's sorry, but she's done with me. She says she wants to be with Steve and I need to stay away. I can't believe my ears. My eyes are all teared up, I'm confused, I can't breathe, and my stomach is all knotted up!

Therapist: Have you ever felt these feelings and sensations prior to this time?

Client: Yes.

Therapist: (*with intensity*) Go back, back, back in time to an earlier time, perhaps the very first time that you feel these similar feelings and sensations. First impressions! What's happening now?

Client: I'm terrified, Mommy and my sister are driving away from the house, and they're leaving me! What am I going to do? They're leaving me all alone!

Therapist: What are you feeling now?

Client: (*emoting*) I'm scared to death, they're leaving me. My heart is racing, my breath is erratic, and I've got that knot in my stomach. What am I going to do?

Therapist: Have you ever felt these feelings before this moment?

Client: I ah, ah ... (*stumbling for words*)

Therapist: Are these old feelings that you are familiar with or new feelings and sensations that you've never experienced before?

Client: I've felt this way before.

Step Six

We are now reaching the ISE:

Therapist: Go back, back, back in time to an earlier time, perhaps the very first time you feel these feelings and sensations!

Client: I, I, I can't see anything.

Therapist: Not see, what's happening now, indoors or out?

Client: I don't know, I, I … (*The client demonstrates some hesitancy to move ahead.*)

Therapist: (*Tapping client on the forehead*) Back, back to that time that you know is the first time you feel these feelings and sensations, that knot in your stomach, the shortness of breath. Be there now! Indoors or out?

Client: It's dark. I'm scared! I can't move! I'm stuck! I feel trapped!

Therapist: What's happening now?

If the client hadn't responded to the tap on the forehead, the therapist might have chosen to tell the client to make up a story. In the client's mind there is often a knowing that the next step will be uncomfortable, so they may try to hesitate. When the client begins to make up the story it helps to keep them in their subconscious (the conscious mind does not make up stories). As the client begins making up the story, the subconscious is actually going into the real scenario. At about that time, the client usually has an "Aha! Experience" and realizes that this is not a fabrication at all. The therapist can just say, "Make up a story about what might have happened," or say, "Once upon a time," and let them fill in the rest. I know this may seem like iffy territory, but it has been very effective.

Client: I, I, I … must be getting born. Something is wrong! I must be stuck somehow!

Therapist: What are you feeling?

Client: I'm scared! I've got that knot in my stomach! Oh! Oh! I'm out, but something is wrong. People are rushing around. People are yelling orders at one another! Where's my mommy? I want my mommy! They're taking me away! Where's my mommy! They take me off to another room. I'm in some kind of enclosure. I've got tubes and things sticking out of me! I'm scared!

Therapist: Have you ever noticed these feelings and sensations prior to this time?

Client: No, I've never felt like this before.

Step Seven

Transforming the negative incident:

Therapist: Take a deep breath and imagine this scene happening over again only in a whole, new, better way, a healthier way that works better for you.*

This is the beginning of the transformational piece (reframing). At this point, the therapist should encourage a few possibilities: "This [health issue or complication] is resolved prior to the birth experience. Or perhaps it is resolved by having different parents, or more educated parents." Or, often, I will bring in the adult self, especially if the client needs to be rescued from other adults or situations. Information gathered during the intake portion will help the therapist to give some possibilities. The therapist should never lead the client by giving him or her just one possible solution. The therapist may think he or she knows the best possible outcome for this situation, but they could well be wrong. By giving the client a few options, they will get the idea of where they best need to go for their own healing. When the client arrives at their own solution, they are more likely to embrace it, even if it is the same solution the therapist would have suggested. "Perhaps whatever has caused these difficulties with your birth is taken care of prior to this time. Maybe your mother chooses to do HypnoBirthing instead and avoids these complications altogether, or perhaps you have different parents altogether." This could be thought of as a leverage technique, where the mind tends to choose the more appealing scenario to operate from. After the session the mind can recall both events; it just tends to go with the more appealing version.

---

*This is what Dave Elman referred to as "substitute cause." Elman was not in favor of using substitute causes, but I think he may have based that on conscious thinking and, of course, regression therapy was still in its infancy at that time.

Client: It's just before I get born. The doctors are doing something to manipulate my position. They get me turned around. I'm no longer tangled in the cord.

Therapist: What happens next?

Client: I'm moving down the birth canal. It's tight, but I'm moving. It feels better this time. I'm not scared like before.

Therapist: Now what?

Client: I'm coming out! People are helping, it feels much better somehow. There's my mommy! She's reaching out for me. She holds me close to her, it feels warm and safe. I'm starting to nurse. (*The client is curling and snuggling in the recliner.*)

Therapist: What are you feeling now?

Client: I feel safe and protected; I feel comfortable.

Therapist: Where do you notice these sensations in your body?

Client: In my stomach.

Therapist: Place your hand right there on your stomach, right where you notice these comfortable safe feelings. (*This helps to create the kinesthetic anchor for use later.*) Notice these good feelings of comfort and protection; notice these good feelings building right there beneath your hand; just notice these good feelings growing right there beneath your hand. Anytime you place your hand on your stomach in this manner you notice these good feelings growing right there beneath your hand. Now take a deep breath and breathe all of these good feelings and sensations deep into every cell of your body. (*If we did not do any of this transforming part the client might still experience the necessary healing just by experiencing the circumstances or origin of their issue. That's also the way change was accomplished by some therapists in the past.*)

Client: (*Takes a deep breath*)

Therapist: That's right.

Step Eight

Now we are going back to transform the SSEs, SPE, or SIEs that we have uncovered along the way (Step Five). If there are a lot of these, or if time is short, then just do the most significant scenes and move on. Sometimes I will bring scenes into this process that were not part of the trance work, but were mentioned in the intake portion and seemed to be of great significance. Step Eight and Step Nine help to lead the mind down the merry path, as I like to call it. Because one positive thing happens, it follows that so will another.

Therapist: Now take a deep breath and allow yourself to drift back to the time when you are four years old and your mom and sister are driving away in the car, and imagine this scene happening over in a whole, new, healthier, better way that works better for you, and tell me what's happening.

Client: I wake up from my nap when I hear the front door close. I look outside and see Mom's car pulling away. Mom sees me looking out the front door and backs the car up. She says they're just going down the street to drop my sister off at the neighbor's and she didn't want to wake me up. I jump in the car and ride down the street with Mom.

Therapist: How does that make you feel?

Client: I feel good.

Therapist: Now take a deep breath and breathe these good feelings into every cell of your body. (*This helps to anchor good feelings. It's not necessary to use a kinesthetic anchor for every positive feeling, just the most significant ones.*)

Therapist: Now take a deep breath and feel yourself drifting back, back to the time when your girlfriend, Judy, is with Steve and imagine this scene happening over in a whole, new, healthier way, a way that works better for you. Tell me what's happening now.

Client: I've got a lot more self-confidence now. I realized what Judy was really like a long time ago. I broke it off with her and I've been dating Sally. Sally is really sweet. When I see Judy and Steve together it's no big deal; they deserve each other.

Therapist: How does that make you feel?

Client: I feel fine. It's like no big deal. I'm just happy to be with Sally.

Therapist: Now take a deep breath and breathe these good feelings deep into every cell of your body.

Client: (*Takes a deep breath*)

Therapist: Now allow yourself to drift back to the time that you're flying to Seattle, that December of '98 just after your marriage, and imagine this scene happening over in a whole, new, better way.

Client: I'm flying to Seattle and there is a lot of turbulence. I'm so preoccupied with thoughts of my new bride and getting back for Christmas that I hardly notice.

Therapist: How does that make you feel?

Client: I feel great. All I notice are the good feelings about my new wife and our life ahead of us.

Therapist: Now take a deep breath and breathe these good feelings deep into every cell of your body.

Step Nine

Future Progression or Mental Rehearsal:

This is where the therapist takes the client ahead into the future, most likely to a situation that would normally be emotionally charged for the client, such as that next business trip to Chicago. The future progression, or mental rehearsal, not only helps to lead the mind further along the merry path, it also helps us to know if the work we have just done is successful.

Therapist: Take a deep breath and feel yourself moving ahead in time to next Thursday when you're leaving for Chicago.

Client: I'm driving to the airport. I've been looking forward to this trip. I'll be making a business deal that could be very lucrative. My wife and I have been talking about having kids and this business deal could make things a lot easier on us.

Therapist: What else?

Client: I walk down the concourse to board the plane. Wow! It's like no big deal. I'm still looking forward to the trip. I'm excited about the business deal and having a family. It feels good to get in my seat on the plane. I know I can just sit back and relax. I've got some reading to catch up on and it's like no time at all and the plane is landing in Chicago.

Therapist: How does that make you feel?

Client: I feel great. I know I can fly with ease now.

Therapist: That's right; you can fly with ease now. Now breathe in these good feelings into every cell of your body.

Client: (*Takes a deep breath*)

Oftentimes when I'm working with a phobia, I will encourage another Step Nine in which I actually do lead my client. In this case, I might suggest that as the plane takes off it keeps getting smaller and smaller until soon my client is riding in one of those little kiddy planes from the amusement park. The client is much too big for the plane and their knees are sticking way up. The wind is blowing (maybe they have one of those Snoopy and the Red Baron scarves on). The client zooms around through the sky until they see the airport and zoom in for a landing. As the client makes a perfect three-point landing, a crowd is quickly gathering. A red carpet is rolled out and camera flashes from news reporters are going off. A marching band is playing as a big limousine pulls up. The mayor gets out and gives the client a big key to the city, and congratulates the client for being the first person to successfully pilot one of these kiddy planes cross country. The client is swept up in the limousine and taken away. The subconscious mind seems to like these ridiculous images and hangs on to them. I've had some interesting experiences with these images.

If the client fails to have a positive future progression, it's not a good sign. Often this means that we either didn't get to the ISE or we may have missed something of importance in the ISE. The necessity for another regression is likely. Although I have been surprised that many times the regression ended up being successful after all, I recommend being positive no matter what. It's important to use good hypnotic language at the end of the session, so as not to undermine the helpful work you have just done.

It's always helpful to give the client some good posthypnotic suggestions based on the regression, prior to emerging them from trance. *You can just sit back and relax*, or *You can fly with ease now*, is some positive verbiage the client used during the trance session.

Using a client's own words to feed back to them has a real power to it. You might notice the therapist parroted back, *You can fly with ease now,* right after the client said it. This is a quick, easy way to start compounding their own positive suggestions. There is a real power in using the client's own words. Be aware, though, that if you do it every single time it can seem annoying, so use good judgment.

After emerging the client from trance, get feedback about their session. What the client experiences in trance will have a lot more detail than we as therapists will be aware of. Also, they need to express their new-found feelings. Perhaps they experienced some epiphany that we weren't aware of. Have the client test the anchor that they were given in trance. In this case the therapist would have the client place a hand on their stomach and notice those new good feelings.

Therapist: Place your hand on your stomach just like you did a moment ago.

Client: (*Places hand on stomach*)

Therapist: Now, notice those good feelings of being safe and comfortable; feel them building right there beneath your hand.

Client: (*Nods that he notices the sensations*)

Therapist: Any time you want to feel these comforting feelings and sensations, all you have to do is place your hand on your stomach in this manner, as you are right now. So, in any situation where you want to feel these good feelings and sensations (not just when flying in airplanes), all you need to do is place your hand on your stomach just in this manner. (*Avoid saying things like when you get on a plane, or feel fear of airplanes. These are painted statements and could place doubt in the mind of your client and undermine the good work that you have just done.*)

Step Ten

Check in with your client. Ask them what they noticed. The client is experiencing things that we as therapists are not always aware of. The client may have had some epiphany that wasn't apparent to the therapist, so allow those things to come out and support them. Let them express what they need to, and this will help them to integrate the session into their lives.

Give your client an action plan based on what has happened during the regression. In the case of fear of flying, its best if the client is getting on the plane first thing in the morning. If not, I tell them to drive out to the airport and watch the planes and visit the terminal as much as possible. This will convince them that the work we have just done has been effective.

Will more sessions be necessary? This is a dicey area. In the above example, the client's therapy is successfully completed. If the therapist were to suggest further sessions at this time, it could plant doubt in his mind and undermine the good work we have just done (very anti-hypnotic). The therapist must seem positive and confident about the session so as not to place doubt in the client's mind. I know some therapists are used to working within (and selling blocks of) six sessions or six months or however many. Some of this may be valid for certain issues and some of it may be to keep a more stable flow of income for the therapist. We all need to make a living; however, I never base the number of sessions on how much money I need to make and I see more clients and am busier than any other therapist in my area. The only time that we sell package deals to clients is in the area of weight loss, due to the nature of that issue.

Many clients come to me for just one session, especially for smoking. Occasionally, I will suggest we do an evaluation in two weeks or so (for some issues) and I do some compounding at that time. This method has worked well for me and doesn't tend to place any doubt in the client's mind. Most of us have been to a doctor for something and we were asked to come back for an evaluation at some later time. This seems like normal procedure to the client. If the client in our example was not leaving for his next plane trip for several months, I would have suggested a follow-up just prior to his next flight. I do this not because the hypnosis wasn't successful, but because in that amount of time there are too many opportunities for the hypnosis to be undermined. If someone else started talking to the client about his past fear of flying, they could eventually convince his subconscious mind that it is still a problem. Through the use of simple suggestion work in the follow-up session, we can guard against such things and compound the positive things we've already achieved.

I have done many regressions similar to the above example. Not every regression goes smoothly or follows the layout of this plan as closely. The skill of the therapist will help keep the process moving along nicely. There could be many SSEs or SIEs. The transformational piece could take off in many directions. It's good to know that, as the therapist, you don't have to come up with all of the answers. Our clients' subconscious minds know the source of the issue and how to solve it. It's up to the therapist to simply guide the client through his or her own process.

I hope that through this example it has become more obvious that the issue the client comes in with may not have anything to do with the cause of their distress (in this case a fear of flying). If the therapist had bought into flying in airplanes as the only possible cause of the issue, the client may still be stuck with their phobia. In this case, even though I didn't spell it out in the session, the client's phobia had its basis in the birth experience. The fears of being stuck in the birth canal (possible claustrophobia) and being separated from his mother right away (possible abandonment), along with having the cord wrapped around his neck and being a breech birth were all the origins of feelings that became triggered by flying on airplanes. When we board an airplane, we're giving up control to the flight crew and the equipment. For most people this doesn't present a big problem. However, for someone with control issues this can be significant. The worst driver in the world with control issues will feel safer behind the wheel of a car than as a passenger, even though that control is an illusion. In the case of our fellow with fear of flying, he also had to deal with issues of abandonment that were being brought to the forefront by being away from his new bride.

An abbreviated version of these ten steps is provided in the Appendix for use as a protocol to follow while doing a session. This is for the use of skilled hypnotherapists only.

Let's take another look at our row of dominoes in relation to this last regression (see Figure 8).

I'm going to give another example of a recent regression. This was a Transformational Replay done by a pair of my students. I wanted to use this as an example because it was very concise and had some nice elements to it. The student therapist did a really nice job; however, the transcript is not quite word for word. I was at times whispering in the student therapist's ear to give advice, and to report that here would only serve to make the transcript a bit confusing. Therefore, I have taken some liberty to smooth out the wording for simplicity. The session only hits on two SSEs before getting to the ISE, and this really simplifies the regression and makes for an easy example. Often a session would hit more SSEs.

During the intake portion of the session we find that our student client struggles with anxiety, low confidence, self-doubt, and withdraws a lot. She reports having a hard time speaking up or giving her opinion. She reports that her anxiety is pretty constant and even getting ready for class today brings it up. Having to perform in some way or talking to adults makes it even worse.

Our student therapist is doing a good job of taking the client to her special place and on to a happy carefree time. I will begin the dialogue after that point.

Therapist: Go back, back in time to a recent time, perhaps the most recent time, that you notice these feelings of anxiety. Take a deep breath and be there now. What's happening now?

Client: It's just this morning. I'm out feeding my mare. I'm going to be taking her with me when I move out of state. Dad won't want me to; he wants to keep a horse around. It was my brother's horse. He'll want me to take this mare with me.

Therapist: How does that make you feel?

Client: I feel anxious, nervous.

Figure 8
Dominoes for Fear of Flying Example

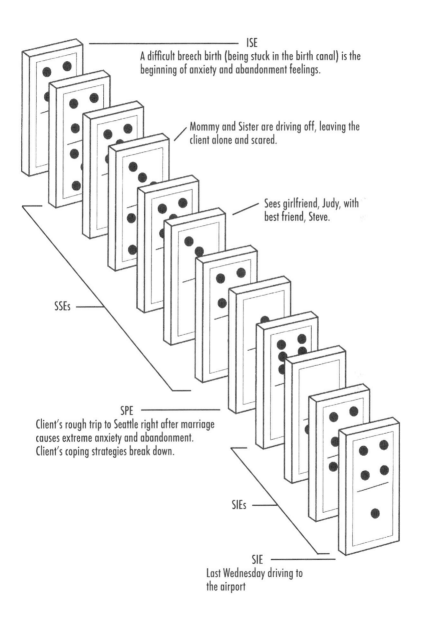

ISE

A difficult breech birth (being stuck in the birth canal) is the beginning of anxiety and abandonment feelings.

Mommy and Sister are driving off, leaving the client alone and scared.

Sees girlfriend, Judy, with best friend, Steve.

SSEs

SPE

Client's rough trip to Seattle right after marriage causes extreme anxiety and abandonment. Client's coping strategies break down.

SIEs

SIE

Last Wednesday driving to the airport

Therapist: Take a deep breath and feel yourself moving back, back to an earlier time, when you feel the same feelings and sensations. Tell me what's happening now?

Client: I'm in the kitchen, its dark in the kitchen. Mom is in the hall. I'm hiding under the table (*client is emoting*), but she'll find me. She grabs me by the arm and jerks me and slaps me; her eyes are scary. Mom hears Dad and she stops.

Therapist: How does that make you feel?

Client: It feels better now. She won't do anything if Dad is around.

Therapist: Go back, back in time to an earlier time, when you feel these familiar feelings and sensations.

Client: I'm a few months old. She's (*Mom*) holding me. I'm scared. She's trying to feed me, but she's mad and doesn't want to, but she doesn't want anyone else to feed me either. She's mad at me, cause I'm here. She's pregnant with my brother, but she doesn't know it yet. I don't like to eat with her; she's rough and she forces me to eat. I just go ahead and eat because I can't get away. I don't want to eat that much, I do it to not make her mad.

Therapist: How does that make you feel?

Client: I feel anxious, scared.

Therapist: Have you ever felt these feelings and sensations prior to this time?

Client: No, this is the first time.

Therapist: Do you make any decisions at this moment?

Client: I'm bad, I'm very bad. I've ruined her life. I have to be really good and quiet and stay out of the way.

Therapist: (*Beginning transformational piece*) Imagine this scene starting over, just like rewinding a tape. This time imagine this scene happening over in a whole, new, healthier way—a way that works better for you. Tell me what's happening now.

Client: (*Even though the therapist did not suggest it, the student client knows enough to bring her adult self into the scene.*) Adult Self comes into the scene. Adult Self loves babies. Adult Self holds and feeds baby client gently. Adult Self trusts baby to know when she has had enough. It feels warm, there's purple and blue and calm.

Therapist: (*Giving the client a pillow and allowing the client to hug the pillow (baby client) and comfort the baby, taking in all the good feelings.*) How does that make you feel?

Client: I feel calm, I feel safe, I feel great.

Therapist: Where do you notice these good feelings and sensations in your body?

Client: I feel it right here in my chest.

Therapist: That's right. Place your hand on your chest just like you are doing and feel the good feelings building right there beneath your hand. Feel the good, calm, safe feelings building right there beneath your hand. Any time you wish to feel these good, calm, safe feelings and sensations, just place your hand on your chest, just in this manner. Now take a deep breath and allow yourself to move back to the scene where you are under the table in the kitchen, and imagine this scene happening over in a whole, new, healthier way, a way that works better for you. Tell me what's happening now.

Client: Adult Self comes into the kitchen. She gets into Mom's face and tells her off. She tells Mom to be nice and not to hit. Let Little Client be herself. Mom knows Adult Self is right. Mom shrinks down and Adult Self is big.

Therapist: How does that make you feel?

Client: I feel strong. I feel like my feet are solid on the ground. I'm a good girl. I can say no. Adult Self talks to little brother in the crib and tells him she's his friend and is there to help him. He trusts Adult Self now. He knows it will be better for him and everyone else now.

Therapist: How does that make you feel?

Client: I feel great. I feel safe.

Therapist: Now take a deep breath and feel yourself moving into the future and tell me what is different now.

Client: I'm talking with my dad about the mare. I feel confident. Things are going much more smoothly than I had imagined. He wants to have a horse around the place. It doesn't have to be the mare. I tell him I'll take good care of her. My brother will probably bring another horse over anyway.

Therapist: How does that make you feel?

Client: Wow, I feel so much more confident; things are going better now.

Therapist: Now take in a deep breath and breathe in these good feelings into every cell of your body and feel yourself sinking deeper and deeper. You can allow yourself to sink as deeply as you desire for I won't be asking any more questions and you can sink as deeply as you desire. (*The therapist gives some positive suggestions around what has just occurred and emerges the client from trance.*)

After emerging:

Therapist: What are you noticing?

Client: I never remembered any of that stuff. The eating stuff relates to me now. I eat when I don't even feel like it and just to make other people happy. When my grandparents were around, Mom wouldn't let them feed me. I remember being so little and powerless. I've done that hiding thing and not speaking up as a result. I could feel the texture of the table legs and the linoleum on my knees. I could have moved along faster and the therapist's voice worked well.

Even though this was the student therapist's first attempt at doing a regression, she did a pretty good job. I offered some input and there were some fine points that got skipped over, but all in all it went really well. While our client had been aware of her anxiety, she had managed to function using her coping strategies—things like withdrawing, being quiet, and avoiding uncomfortable situations. She may never have experienced an SPE the way I have spelled it out in the text, and that is not so unusual. A person wouldn't necessarily have to experience that symptom-producing event to want to heal themselves.

The fact that the client was also a student and had a good knowledge of the process helped out. Typically, clients wouldn't bring in the adult self without some help from the therapist.

When the therapist got the client in touch with a recent time that she felt the anxiety (Step Four in your Transformational Replay guide), it worked out well for this particular client. Most of time the therapist will need to be a bit more thorough at getting the client in touch with their feelings. This step is done to create the affect bridge and we need to make the most of this opportunity. If we don't get the client fully in touch with her feelings, the regression could fizzle. It would have been helpful for the client to describe the feelings and sensations a bit more, especially the body sensations that are associated with the feelings.

When the therapist got the client back to the first SSE that came up (under the kitchen table) (Step Five in your replay guide), the client began emoting and getting into the feelings. Soon Dad's presence became apparent and those feelings shifted tremendously. The therapist was able to move the regression to the next step successfully. However, if you are in a scene where the feelings of the scene shift dramatically, you can lose the affect bridge. If that happens the safe thing to do is to back the scene up just prior to Dad becoming apparent, so that the client is back in the feelings of anxiety (affect bridge) and then move ahead to next scene. This can save a lot of time and struggle.

When the ISE was reached (Step Six in your guide), I wasn't totally convinced that it *was* the ISE for a few reasons. First, the fear around this scene came up really fast—almost before it got started. This may be an indicator that the fear had a beginning in a similar situation prior to this time. Also, the client talked of Mother not allowing anyone else to feed her, yet there is no indication of anyone else in the scene. This might indicate an earlier experience of this type of feeding scene. The client also said that she doesn't like to eat with her mother, which again could indicate an earlier experience of this nature. The client seemed very certain that this was the first time that she had experienced these feelings. Pushing the regression back further may have brought out another scene or just reaffirmed that this really is the ISE.

When the therapist asks the client what decisions she makes (great!), the client comes up with, *I'm bad, I'm very bad. I have to be really good and quiet and stay out of the way.* This is the type of decision that is made at an early time and follows us through life. The decision that "I'm bad, I'm very bad," creates shame in an individual. When shame occurs it means that there is something inherently wrong. This is different from "I have done a bad thing." (This can be fixed.) With shame, a person feels there is something deficient in his or her being. This creates low self worth and other problems just like this client has been experiencing. This will translate into a huge shift in this person's aliveness.

Another huge piece that came out of this scene was the piece around eating. The client learned early on to just ignore her own body signals and eat anyway to avoid causing a problem. Her own words were, *I don't want to eat that much; I do it to not make her mad.* I'm sorry to say that a lot of us learned to overeat early on and this is an extreme example of how that can occur. The overeating issue had not come up in the interview; however, it would have been easy for the therapist to say, *And has this decision affected you in some way?* If the light hadn't already come on for the client, that statement would help to flip the switch. In this case, the client did make that connection. As she came out of trance the first thing she said was, "I never remembered that stuff. That eating stuff all relates to me right now."

This did get discussed as part of her action plan. There are a number of ways that the therapist might help the client to incorporate new eating behaviors into her life. Simply saying, *Just notice the changes around your eating habits from now on,* may be all it takes, especially since in the transformative piece the client fed the baby herself and took charge of that. Or you might try something like, *When you're eating, allow the presence of Grandmother to comfort you* (since she had referred to Grandmother and being fed during the session). Another approach is to ask the client, "How will you notice the new changes in your life?" This is a good approach because the client is coming up with his or her own action plan.

During the reframing portion (relates to Step Seven in your guide), the client brought in her adult self to take control in this scene. Since the client was also one of our students, she had been through the inner child portion of the training and it was a natural transition for her. Another client may not make that connection. Whenever the child is at risk it is good to suggest that the adult self can come in to take control of this scene. This will help to put the client in control in their everyday life.

Within this transformative portion the client refers to feeling warm, purple and blue, calm. I've heard some therapists say things like, *Purple is not a feeling, or depression is not a feeling, or avoidance is not a feeling. Describe your feelings.* We are dealing with the subconscious. If your client is in a feeling state, then purple or some other term probably does have meaning for them as a feeling. It doesn't matter if the therapist is unable to know exactly what that means to the client. If the client says that they are feeling something and they are not obviously in avoidance, then accept that what they say is a feeling, is a feeling. If we question it, we are likely to get the conscious mind involved.

Moving back through (Step Eight in your guide) and reframing the SSEs that were uncovered along the way, we see that this process went quite smoothly. That is often the case. Once the client has done the transformative piece, they tend to move through the rest more easily. At one point, she even brings in some healing around her little brother.

The future progression (Step Nine of your guide) went right to the piece that had been discussed in the client's most recent experience of anxiety (Step Four in your guide). The client was comfortable now and able to talk with her dad about taking the mare with her. How we approach things (from the very essence of who we are) has a huge influence on the outcome. Let's say I want to approach the president of my company about a promotion. If I go into the president's office as the guy with no self-confidence, someone who has been turned down for every raise or promotion that has ever come along, and someone who really feels like they are undeserving of anything more challenging than being the mail clerk, what am I likely to end up with? On the other hand, if I walk into the president's office with my head high, confident, and knowing that I'm the best possible choice for this new position, the likely outcome will be much more positive. The client in the Transformational Replay example has likely avoided confrontation in the past or has had a low expectation of the possible outcome. With her newfound confidence, she's likely to approach confrontation as the deserving, intelligent individual that I know her to be.

The last part of the Transformational Replay (Step Ten)—the check-in with the client—went smoothly. The client said right away that she wanted to go play in the water. There was nothing about water in the session; however, playing in the water likely has inner child significance to the client. Earlier I mentioned some possible action plans around the eating issues that were uncovered. Other possibilities might involve being with the horse or spending time with her little brother. The possibilities are only limited by the creativity of the therapist and client.

The following is another example of a Transformational Replay that I just did recently. This example involves a gentleman with a fear of public speaking, that I had been working with. This client is a highly intelligent, self-motivated and successful individual. His business requires him to speak in front of groups and conduct meetings on a regular basis. He has been able to do the speaking as necessary, but has never been comfortable with it. He also feels as though he has not been as effective as he could be, due to his nervousness.

As I mentioned earlier, I usually start with simpler methods (suggestion work) before moving into Transformational Replay. I had done other work with this client and it had been helpful, but he was still having difficulties. My client was doing all of the right things, such as not avoiding speaking situations, and he even joined Toastmasters. This client had been managing fairly well until he found out that he would have to give the toast at his brother's upcoming wedding. We could think of this moment as his SPE, since the upcoming event caused the old fears to come back in a big way and the usual coping strategies did not seem to be enough. When the client thought of the upcoming event he would notice nervousness, fear, and sensations in the pit of his stomach. I didn't use a SUDs level in this instance. I did, however, notice his body language. This client normally seems quite calm, although when we would talk of the upcoming ceremony I would notice his feet twitching.

Even though I had worked with this client before, we had never done any interactive process. So I explained how interacting would be different. I also told him that I might be tapping him on the forehead at some point during the session and that this would be to engage the subconscious mind. I also explained that I might at some point ask him to make up a story and told him how this would also engage the subconscious mind.

This client easily achieved somnambulism and after going to his safe place at the beach we regressed back to the happy, carefree, active time. This is a time when he's twelve years old and playing ice hockey with all of his friends. Again, this is done to show the client that they can regress back in a non-threatening way. It also provides the scene that we can use for systematic desensitization, if necessary. We will pick up the dialogue from here.

Therapist: In a moment I'm going to ask you to go back in time, and you will go back in time, back to a recent time, perhaps the most recent time, that you had difficulties speaking in front of a group. Take a deep breath and be there now. What's happening now?

Client: I'm at the Toastmasters meeting. I have a job as the timekeeper. I'm called up to describe my duties and it should be quite simple. I feel like others can see that I'm nervous and that's making it worse. I'm able and anxious to finish and sit down.

Therapist: How does that make you feel?

Client: I feel anxious; I feel fear.

Therapist: Where do you notice these sensations in your body?

Client: I feel it in my gut and in my chest, even my head. It's anxiety, it's uncomfortable, like impending doom.

Therapist: That's right, now take a deep breath and feel yourself drifting back, back in time to an earlier time, when you feel these feelings of anxiety, the sensations in your gut and chest. Moving back and be there now. What's happening now?

Client: I'm in college giving a report on the free trade agreement. It's a group project and it's my turn. I'm reading what I have written verbatim. I'm just not comfortable and I come across very scripted.

Therapist: How does that make you feel?

Client: It's those same feelings in my stomach and chest. There's a lack of confidence and it gets worse with each passing moment of my turn. It's hideous.

Therapist: Take a deep breath and feel yourself drifting back, back in time to an earlier time, when you feel these same feelings and sensations in your stomach and chest, the fear, the anxiety. Be there now, what's happening now? (*This statement is made with some force and intention behind it.*)

Client: I'm in high school, speaking in front of my English class. I'm nervous as I start out, but it gets better. Moving into the presentation, I'm getting nervous and I feel the body sensations. I'm able to speak about the subject somewhat.

Therapist: What are you feeling?

Client: A lot of fear. I'm afraid of what others will think if I screw up.

Therapist: (*Since the client was obviously in the feeling and in the moment, I just pushed him back more directly, as I sometimes will do.*) Go back, back, back to an earlier time when you feel these same feelings and sensations.

Client: I'm ten years old or so and with some friends. A group of guys are ganging up on me, verbally. They are trying to belittle me. I feel anger and frustration, hurt, I'm unsure of how to fight back and respond verbally.

Therapist: Go back, back in time to an earlier time that you feel these similar feelings and sensations. Be there now. What's happening now?

Client: It's an argument with me and my mother. There's some name calling. I'm seven or eight years old. I'm being verbally assaulted, cussed at out of anger.

Therapist: How does that make you feel?

Client: I feel frustrated, angry.

Therapist: Go back; back in time to an earlier time, perhaps the very first time, you feel these feelings and sensations. Be there now. What's happening now?

Client: I'm riding in the car. I'm on my way to go get a shot. I'm three years old. My uncle is there and he's calling me a baby. I'm very angry with him. I'm not a baby. I don't want anyone sticking me with a needle. My parents are in the car. I'm pissed off.

Therapist: Go back, back in time to an earlier time, perhaps the very first time you feel these feelings and sensations. Tell me what's happening. What's happening now?

Client: A, ah … (*brief hesitation*).

Therapist: I'm going to tap you on the forehead. (*I tap the client's forehead as I continue to speak.*) Go back, back in time to an earlier time that you feel these same feelings and sensations, those sensations in your stomach and chest, perhaps you're pissed, angry, fearful. What's happening; what's happening now?

Client: I'm very, very young. My real father is in the room; I haven't seen him since I was a little baby. He's yelling hateful things. I've never met him, only heard about him from Mother's description.

Therapist: How does that make you feel?

Client: I feel worthless. I feel deep, emotional hurt.

Therapist: Do you make some decision at this point?

Client: There must be something wrong with me to be the recipient of all this negativity.

Therapist: What are you feeling?

Client: I feel the anger and frustration.

Therapist: Where do you notice these feelings in your body?

Client: In the pit of my stomach, like before.

Therapist: Have you ever noticed these feelings and sensations prior to this time?

Client: No, I've never had these feelings before. This is the first time.

Therapist: Now take a deep breath and feel yourself relax. Now just imagine this whole scene starting over, just like rewinding a tape. Now imagine this scene happening over in a whole, new, healthier, better way, a way that works better for you. In fact, you may want to bring your adult self in to take control in this scene. So imagine this scene happening over in a whole, new, healthier way, a way that works better for you, and tell me what's happening.

Client: I'm (*adult self*) responding with my own assault and defending myself.

Therapist: Is Little Client aware of what's happening?

Client: Yes, Little Client is aware.

Therapist: How does that feel?

Client: Feels protected and cared for. Adult Client is comforting him and making him safe. It feels much better.

Therapist: Is there anything else that needs to happen here to make Little Client feel better?

Client: No, Little Client is doing just fine now.

Therapist: Would it be okay to hug Little Client?

Client: Yes, he wants that.

Therapist: I'm going to give you a pillow (*as I place a pillow on his chest*) and just put your arms around this pillow and hold Little Client close and make him feel safe. Make sure that Little Client can get his ear up against your chest and hear your heart beating so he can tell how sincere you are. How does that make you feel?

Client: I feel protected and cared for.

Therapist: Where do you notice these feelings in your body?

Client: I feel them in my stomach and chest. (*The client places his hands right where he feels the sensations without needing to be encouraged.*)

Therapist: Just notice these good feelings and sensations of being cared for and protected; notice these feelings building right there beneath your hands. Any time you want to feel these good feelings and sensations, all you need to do is just place your hands in this very manner. Now take a deep breath and breathe these good feelings and sensations deep into every cell of your body.

In a moment you will go back to the scene where you and your mother were arguing, and imagine this scene happening over in a whole, new, healthier, better way—a way that works better for you. Tell me what's happening now.

Client: Adult Self is there and it's all turned around. Adult Self is confronting her saying, "What's wrong with you, assaulting someone so young. There's a better way to discipline than to shout obscenities." As a grown up I can turn it all around. (*Client realizes*)

Therapist: How does that make you feel?

Client: It feels like I'm ok and those words are only words. They don't affect who I am.

Therapist: Take a deep breath and breathe these good feelings and sensations deep into every cell of your body. And now just allow yourself to go back to the time when you're in college giving a report. Imagine this scene happening over in a whole, new, healthier way and tell me what's happening.

Client: I'm looking directly at the audience with confidence. I don't even have to read. I know my subject and I engage the audience. I use gestures and body language with confidence and it works well.

Therapist: How does that make you feel?

Client: I feel empowered. I feel confident. It feels good. I feel good.

Therapist: Now take a deep breath and breathe in all of these good feelings and sensations deep into every cell of your body. Now just move back to that recent time when you are addressing the Toastmasters meeting. Imagine this scene happening over in a whole, new, healthier way, a way that works better for you, and tell me what's happening now.

Client: I had no worry the night before and slept well and feel refreshed. It's no big deal. I'm able to bond with my audience and I relate to the job and am done with it. There's no need for fear to explain something so basic. My audience shows their appreciation.

Therapist: How does that make you feel?

Client: I feel empowered and accepted.

Therapist: Now take a deep breath and breathe these good feelings and sensations deep into every cell of your body. Now just allow yourself to move ahead into the future at your brother's wedding and tell me what's happening now.

Client: I'm getting up and asking for everyone's attention. I feel like I have something to say. I'm not sure of exactly everything I'm going to say, but I know it will go ok. I'll be honest and speak from the heart and move on.

Therapist: How does that make you feel?

Client: I feel confident, only the slightest uneasiness. Mostly it's just a feeling of indifference.

Therapist: Now take a deep breath and breathe in all of these good feelings of confidence deep into every cell of your body and feel yourself sinking deeper. You can allow yourself to sink as deeply as you desire now, for I won't be asking you any more questions and you can sink as deeply as you desire. (*At this point I give the client some positive suggestions based on what has just occurred.*)

After emerging from trance:

Therapist: What are you noticing?

Client: I feel much better, more confident.

Therapist: That's right. Now place your hands on your stomach and chest once again. (*Client places hands in the same manner as before.*) Notice those good feelings building right there beneath your hands. Notice the good feelings of being protected and cared for. Notice these good feelings building right there beneath your hands. Do you notice the good feelings there beneath your hands?

Client: Yes, I do notice them.

Therapist: Any time you want to feel these good feelings and sensations, just place your hands in this very manner and you will feel these good feelings of being protected and cared for.

Client: (*Nods his acknowledgment*) A lot of it I remembered consciously. I didn't remember any of that stuff as an infant. I never remembered my father, but I heard of things that he had said and done.)

This regression is a good example because it is a common issue that is likely to occur in your office fairly often. Also, this regression had six SSEs that we visited, which is more customary than our previous example. This session moved very smoothly and quickly. The client always remained in the present tense and in the moment. There was not a lot of emoting in this session (some tearing at most); however, body language played a big role. You might recall me talking about his feet moving nervously during the intake whenever we talked about the wedding. During the future progression, I noticed his feet remained calm.

You may have noticed that when we reached the ISE, there was again a decision made (somewhat similar to the previous example), where the client feels he's worthless, has deep emotional hurt, and thinks there must be something wrong with him. As in the previous example, these are the kinds of decisions that create shame. It isn't that he has done something wrong; it's that there is something fundamentally wrong with him and he's worthless. Again, if the client has done something wrong, that thing can change. This is a lot different from having some inherent flaw that is unlikely to be changed. If you noticed on the return trip through the ISEs and reframing the incident with his uncle, the client said, "I'm okay." It's not that the client was saying I'm okay—as in things are copasetic; but that I'm okay as an individual and there is nothing inherently wrong with me. As the therapist listening to the client's words and noticing the subtleties of inflection and body language, it's easier to pick up on that than through the printed word. However, this is a big thing that demonstrates overcoming that shame piece that was present earlier.

You may have noticed in the future progression piece that the client feels confident making the toast. He did express just a little uneasiness and this is normal. I wouldn't expect anyone—even someone who had no problems speaking in front of large groups—to achieve a one on the SUDs level. A certain amount of stress would be present for anyone in that situation. It's similar with fear of flying. Even a seasoned traveler would experience some stress getting through busy airports and boarding crowded planes.

The action plan for this client was fairly easy because he has to speak in front of others on a regular basis. Just noticing how things are different now will help to reassure him for that wedding toast and the future. I encouraged him to be more aware of the inner child and let him come out to play. He was going boating soon and so it was a good time to let the little client be there and interact. I also encouraged him to be more aware of the little client on the job and to interact there.

Oftentimes, the words coming out of the client make sense to the therapist, but are confusing to a reader. In this case, the client used particularly good grammar, which made it easier for me to transfer to print. This example is pretty much word-for-word as I wrote it down.

Conclusion

The examples that I have given are quite linear and that is not only typical as to how a session may occur, but also makes for easier understanding. Sessions don't always go like a script; sometimes the client may jump around in time. As the therapist, just stay calm and go with your client and stick with the feelings.

The feelings that we establish for the affect bridge may seem to change, such as in the last example with public speaking. We started with feelings of nervousness. Those feelings of nervousness translated into fear, then lack of confidence, then frustration, anger, hurt, and finally feelings of worthlessness. These feelings all relate to the same thing. If you'll notice in the text, it was only the description of the feelings that changed, while the body sensations remained the same throughout the regression. This is why it's always good to check in on the body sensations. One might think that they have lost the affect bridge if the description of the feelings changes; however, I've rarely had that actually happen.

Often when a client begins to emote (in or out of trance), the therapist will reach for the box of tissues or want to touch or hug their client. This is not a good idea. If, as the therapist, you offer a tissue or a hug or touch, what is the message that you are giving? What you are saying, without speaking, is, *Now, now, stop crying or feeling that way.* Basically, we are invalidating the client's feelings. Often when the therapist offers a tissue or other support to the client, it's because the therapist is not comfortable with the client's feelings. So the therapist unwittingly is shutting those feelings down. I keep tissues within reach so that the client can grab a tissue if they desire (which is a lot different from me handing the tissues to them). During trance, allow the client to emote and have their feelings (they don't have to stay there for long), and use those feelings (the somatic affect bridge) to keep the session moving. When the session is over you can offer the client a tissue. Some clients that I have worked with previously will grab some tissues before we get started (knowing that they may need them in the session), and that's fine. When the client grabs their own tissues ahead of time, I am not influencing their feelings or actions.

Be sure to keep other necessities at hand, such as a plastic bat and pillows (may be necessary for a Gestalt or inner child piece) and blankets.

During the intake portion it is necessary to explain to the client the difference between the conscious and subconscious minds. It is also necessary to explain the hypnotic process. When explaining to the client that you will be doing a regression, simply tell them that we will be traveling back in time to uncover the origin of their issue (feelings, symptoms). Do not explain the steps of this process to the client. If you explain all of the steps to them you will engage their conscious, analytical mind, and they will be waiting and wondering about each step. Or the session may not follow the steps exactly, causing questions to arise in their mind. In either case, you will likely only achieve a pseudo regression at best. Also, over-explaining the regression or the hypnotic process tends to remove the magic of hypnosis. I have seen hypnotists explain hypnosis to such an extent that they took the magic of hypnosis right out of the client's session. Leave some room in the process for mystery. This allows the subconscious to create miracles.

What if I need to end the session before it is completed? I like to make things as clean as possible and not send the client out of the office with a bunch of half-plowed furrows to think about until our next session. If there is time enough, I will reframe the last SSE that was uncovered and bookmark it. If there's no time to reframe, I will bookmark the session by telling the client that we are out of time and we will return to this very moment (describing the moment with a few words) in our next session. It's amazing how easily a client can pick right up where we left off in the next session.

Why might a session not succeed? If a client wants to be hypnotized and wants to achieve their goal, then that is what will most likely happen. If a client has issues with losing control and is trying to stay conscious and be hypnotized at the same time, it won't work. A person cannot remain vigilant and be hypnotized at the same time. We tell our clients that they are in control and, ultimately, that is so. However, a client needs to relinquish control enough to be hypnotized or we will never get anywhere, no matter how much they desire change. It is up to us as therapists to create the space that will allow the client to go into trance. There are times when it won't happen. It's been necessary to send some clients home, telling them to let me know when they're ready to go into trance (although that is extremely rare). In time that client may return (after having a chance to process things in their mind) to move ahead with their work.

There are other reasons why someone might not succeed, such as secondary gain. It's hard sometimes for us to imagine that someone would not want to make healthy change in his or her life. However, often the payoff for keeping their issue may be bigger than the benefits of healing them. Let's say that if the client's issue were healed they would no longer be able to stay in their parent's mansion and enjoy the maid service. Or certainly it could be something more simple like, *Without this issue I'll lose my pension or I'll have to go back to school or get a job or take care of my family or make love to that husband I can't stand.*

Also, the healing may be of such significance that it would change the very essence of our being. What if the client has survived their whole life by being a victim? It might seem strange that someone would want to continue in this mode if they don't have to, but this is who they are. This has become their identity, their method of survival and without it the big question is, *Who am I? How will I survive?* The truth is they will probably do just fine, but it's frightening to step out into the world with no identity or method to survive. Being the victim is a position of power. It may not be pretty, but it's a way that the individual has learned to manipulate their world. *I can't be expected to do that because of my [fill in the blank]*, or, *Can you take care of this for me because of [fill in the blank]*. Victims get rewarded with charity and favorable judgments. Of course, people do get victimized and people do need to be helped and that's life. The problem in becoming a victim is that we can use that as a position of power. But that also takes away from our ability to have real control in life and to be proactive. You can't take control in your life and move ahead with confidence while maintaining your victimization.

You may have met people who start right off with their victimization as an introduction: *My husband left me six months ago and took all the money from the cookie jar. My sister is in rehab for drugs and I found out she was sleeping with my teenage son when the house caught on fire, cause they sold my TV to get crack so they could deal with the fact that my mother's a born-again alcoholic, overachieving, lesbian, midget pedophile on disability because she shot her foot off trying to hold up a convenience store, because she ran out of gauze for those open sores on her legs, because she was malnourished since that bum cousin of hers fed the food stamps to his stupid coon dog (after all it said food stamps right on the thing) right after she passed out from having sex with him, which gave her those awful warts that kept the reverend from wanting to go down on her every time and that's my loving mother you know, but it's only cause my real daddy, who I am told was a Fuller Brush salesman going from door to door, and that's why I've got this funny hairline thing going on. How about yourself?*

Not all victims talk in run on sentences or are quite as obvious as this example. I have actually been in the process of doing a successful regression with a client and gotten to the ISE, only to notice the client shift at that moment and begin to sabotage their process. The reason for this is that if the client went through the transformative portion, it would mean taking control of their life and taking control would mean giving up their victimization, which in their mind would mean that they would cease to exist.

I have watched a client duck and dodge and go into alternative realities to avoid facing their own healing. I've had them leave and not return to finish their work, even though they are fractions of an inch from achieving their goal. Somewhere in the client's mind it is safer to stick with a survival method that is known to them (even though it's not working that well) than it is to step out into the unknown.

If you think you have gotten to an ISE and your client is expressing feelings of guilt, then it is not the ISE. Guilt is something that had to be learned from a previous experience.

If you are a therapist and you have had training in regression therapy and will be following the methods as I have outlined them here, then I suggest that you relax. Often the therapist becomes fearful of the process because they put too much pressure on themselves. As the therapist you are in the session to help your client find his or her own way. It is not up to you to have the answers. The client already has the answers in their own subconscious mind. Think of your client as a vehicle trying to find its way in the dark. As the therapist you are not the engine, nor are you the steering wheel or tires. You are the headlights that help them find their own way down the road. Remember, the healing always occurs in the recliner in which your client is sitting.

Appendix

The following protocols are not scripts and you cannot expect to use them as scripts. I have had people ask me for my script for doing regression therapy. There is no such thing. If someone did have a script for a regression, it could only lead to a pseudo regression. A true regression cannot be scripted because it's coming from the client and not the therapist. However, protocols will help to keep the therapist on track until the therapist becomes comfortable with the process and can then do it without any aids. When using these protocols I suggest that you never try to read from this book. If a client were to see that you were reading from a book, they might think that you don't have a clue as to what you are doing. If you were being prepped for surgery and the surgeon was thumbing through a medical book looking up spleens, you might feel a bit uneasy yourself.

I suggest that you create your own separate protocol on your word processor using the one in the book as a model. Or you can get a CD of these protocols from Eastburn Hypnotherapy Center at *www.hypnodenver.com*

I also recommend that you put your protocols and any scripts that you use on a regular basis in plastic sheet protectors. Not only does this serve to protect your papers, but also it keeps the pages from rattling and drawing attention to the fact that you are reading from something that has been prepared ahead of time.

Transformational Replay Guide

Step One

Intake, determine session intention.

Step Two

Induction to safe place (stairs work well). Get the client in touch with their senses and anchor good feelings with the breath.

Step Three

This step is done to demonstrate to the client that they can travel back in time and in a non-threatening way.

Take the client back in time to a happy, carefree, active time (this may be your client's point of reference, depending on what you are working on). This needs to be a pleasant experience that we can return to, if necessary.

Step Four

This step starts to move the client back in time toward their ISE, and it's relatively easy because it was just the other day.

Take client to a recent time, perhaps the most recent time, the client had an experience with X. This will most likely be an SIE. Be especially sure to get them in touch with their feelings and find out where they notice these feelings in the body (this will help you to create an affect bridge). There is no need to do the transformational piece until you finish with the ISE.

Step Five

This step will most likely get the client in touch with another SIE, SPE or SSE. Occasionally, a client might go straight to an ISE, but not often. It is likely that you will repeat Step Five a number of times before you get to the ISE.

Take the client back in time to an earlier time that incident "X" occurred or they felt these similar feelings and sensations. (Say, *Take a deep breath and feel yourself drifting back in time, back to an earlier time, perhaps a much earlier time, that "X" occurred, or you felt these similar feelings and sensations.*)

Step Six

You have reached the ISE. (If you're not sure, just ask, *Have you ever felt these feelings or sensations before?* or, *Are these feelings familiar to you, or are these new, unusual feelings?*) Get your client in touch with what's going on here. Abreaction is likely.

Step Seven

Transforming the negative incident:

Often this means bringing in the adult self. Make certain the adult self takes control and that the child is well aware that the adult self is taking charge. Try wording like this: *Let's start this scene over from the beginning, just like rewinding a tape. Imagine this scene happening in a whole, new, healthier, better way, a way that works better for you. You may need to bring in your adult self to take control in this scene.* When the scene has been totally transformed, use a kinesthetic anchor to anchor any good feelings. Ask, *Where do you feel these new, good feelings in your body?*

Step Eight

Now go back and transform the SSEs, SPE, or SIEs that we uncovered along the way (Step Five). If there are a lot of these, or if time is running short, then just do the most important ones and move on.

Step Nine

Future progression:

Take your client ahead into the future, perhaps to a situation that would have been charged for them, like getting on the plane tomorrow.

If you're dealing with a phobia, you may want to run another future progression and make it very ridiculous.

Doing the future progression is an important piece, not just because the client is projecting their new expectations into the future, but also because if the client does not see themselves in the future without their past symptom, then there is probably more work to do. (You probably didn't get to the ISE, or there is more that needs to be cleared.)

Step Ten

Emerging the client from trance:

This step includes emerging your client from trance, checking in with the client, testing the kinesthetic anchor that was given to the client (when necessary), and creating an action plan (homework assignment) for the client.

Inner Child Journey

1. Interview.

2. Induction (use stairs to safe place).

3. Take client on a journey down the path to meet the child. If resistance occurs (*I don't see her on the path*) suggest that there is a curve in the path or a boulder and as soon as we clear that obstacle there is the child.

4. Have the client describe the child (age, clothing, etc.).

5. Is the child aware of the client? Does the child know who the client is? If not, have the client introduce him- or herself to the child. Explain that they are here to protect and play with the child.

6. Tell the client to ask the child what sorts of things the child likes to do (play house, ride bikes, catch pollywogs, etc.). Befriend the child in this manner.

7. Have the client ask the child what sorts of things he or she would like to do together (ride bikes, play on the swings, etc.). It's fine for them to go off and do these things together now.

8. Ask the client if the child and client are ready to hug. The answer will probably be yes. If so, give them a pillow or stuffed animal to hold and feel themselves hugging the child. Ask, *How does that make you feel?*

9. Have the client imagine that their heart is now opening up like a flower and all of the childlike qualities are flowing in from the child through their open heart and into every cell of their body. The child's heart also opens like a flower and all of the client's strengths flow into the child, as well. Now have the two of them meld together as one. Wherever the client goes they now have this new awareness of the child.

10. Use anything that was gleaned from the session to help with an action plan. For example, suggest that the client, between now and the next appointment, go to the park and play on the swings or spend time with a niece or nephew.

If resistance occurs or the child is afraid to play with adult self (*Grandma will hear me and lock me up in the basement*), then an inner child rescue is needed. Regress client to the ISE of Grandmother's abuse and have Adult Self come in to take control of the scene and save the child. Another attempt at a journey should be successful now that the child knows the adult self can be trusted.

References

Hypnotherapy
By Dave Elman
Available through Eastburn Hypnotherapy and Westwood Publishing

Homecoming
By John Bradshaw
Readily available at bookstores
Audio and videocassettes available
P.O. Box 980547
Houston, Texas 77098
(713) 529-9437

For information on workshops and lectures write:
John Bradshaw
2412 South Boulevard
Houston, Texas 77098
Stamped self-addressed envelope required

Answer Cancer
By Stephen C. Parkhill
Omni Hypnosis Publishing
197 Glenwood Road
Deland, Florida 32720

Experimental Hypnosis
By Leslie M. LeCron
Out of print

Gerald F. Kein
Omni Hypnosis
830 North Woodland Boulevard
Deland, Florida 32720
Trainings, tapes, and literature available
www.omnihypnosis.com

Made in the USA
Columbia, SC
24 June 2017